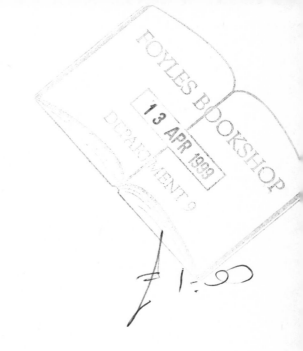

£1.9

The Knee

The Knee

Philippe Segal·Marcel Jacob

Wolfe Medical Publications Ltd

Copyright © Maloine S. A. Éditeur, Paris
(ISBN 2-224-00887-2), 1983
Published in France as 'Le Genou'
English language version published by
Wolfe Medical Publications Ltd, 1984
Printed by Butler and Tanner Ltd,
Frome, Somerset.
ISBN 0 7234 0847 5

This book is one of the titles in the series of
Wolfe Medical Atlases, a series which brings
together probably the world's largest systematic
published collection of diagnostic colour
photographs.
For a full list of Atlases in the series, plus
forthcoming titles and details of our surgical,
dental and veterinary Atlases, please write to
Wolfe Medical Publications Ltd, Wolfe House,
3 Conway Street, London W1P 6HE.

General Editor, Wolfe Medical Atlases:
G. Barry Carruthers, MD(London)

CONTENTS

FOREWORD

Numerous surgical teams have become involved in this study, in France as well as in the rest of the world. We cannot mention them all, but we think we should mention one in particular, giving credit to Albert Trillat and the school at Lyons that he directs. The success of various knee conventions that he has organized attest to his importance.

My collaborator, Philippe Segal MD, 'Professeur Agrégé' studied with him. Subsequently taking to his own wings, Dr Segal became a knee surgeon, particularly active in the field of sports.

Dr Marcel Jacob MD, has been interested in the sports traumatology of the knee and particularly the soccer player for many years now. He is the French Soccer Federation physician and has, of course, been consulted by more than one player on the Rheims team as well as players on teams throughout France.

The backgrounds of these two authors qualify them perfectly for the task of writing this type of text. They were able to express clearly and simply concepts that are occasionally quite complex, using a highly diagrammatic style accompanied by the magnificent illustrations of Professor Bodenschatz

of the Rheims Ecole des Beaux Arts. They were assisted by members of the orthopaedic team of the Rheims University Hospital Centre, which I am proud to have founded. As a result, rheumatologists, surgeons, and physical therapists have contributed to the editing of this book, which, if it is not the only text on the subject, appears to me to be a high quality up-dating that has arrived at the right time.

While the subtitle of this book is sports traumatology, and while it is intended essentially for those involved in sports traumatology and medicine, it is in fact a perfect up-dating on all knee traumatology problems and is consequently of value to all orthopaedic surgeons and physical therapists. The authors did not want to write a treatise (and there is no bibliography with hundreds of references), but rather a text book.

Yves Gerard

Member of the French Academy of Surgery
Professor of Clinical Orthopaedics and Traumatological Surgery at the Rheims University Hospital Centre

PREFACE

This book is particularly intended for surgeons, x-ray specialists, physical therapists, rheumatologists, sports specialists and those in related disciplines, and forms a fundamental element in the instruction of traumatology, physical medicine and physical therapy.

The book was designed by a team of doctors, surgeons and physical therapists at the Rheims University Hospital Centre's Orthopaedics and Traumatology Service. They are:

Professor Jean Jacques Adnet, Head of the Histological Laboratory Service;

Dr Emile Dehoux, Ward Chief;

Dr Marcel Jacob, Rheumatologist, President of the High Commission for the French Soccer Federation (FFF) and instructor at the International Soccer Federation (FIFA);

Mr Bernard Keyser, Physical Therapist and Member of the French Sports Physical Therapy Society (SFKS);

Dr Jean Jacques Lallement, Orthopaedic Surgeon;

Dr Eric Morel, Doctor of Physical Medicine and Consulting Physician for the National Sports and Physical Education Institute (INSEP);

Dr Antoine Pierson, Ward Chief;

Dr Ivan Perringerard, Ward Chief and Assistant Professor of Anatomy;

Dr Mark Raguet, Surgical Intern and Assistant Professor of Anatomy;

Philippe Segal, Professeur Agrégé, Head of Service and Member of the International Society of the Knee (ISK).

The illustrations were done by Rene Bodenschatz, Professor at the Rheims Ecole des Beaux Arts.

We would like to give credit to all of the individuals who, through their work and knowledge of sports medicine, have contributed to the study of the physiology and pathology of the knee, in particular:

J H Aubriot	S Bamas	S Buscayret	R Buillet
P Blaimont	G Bousquet	P Burdin	A Boeda
J Bernageau	J Castaing	P Chambat	J C Chatard
F Commandre	J L Carpentier	J J Comtet	A Durey
H Dejour	Y Demarais	G Demonteil	P Ficat
L P Fischer	J M Ferret	G Forissier	D Goutallier
P Grammont	Y Gerard	J Genety	A Herbert
J J Herbert	J C Imbert	J H Jaeger	I A Kapandji
P Kouvalchouk	M Lequesne	M Lemaire	R Lemaire
J L Lerat	P Maquet	C Mansat	F Mazas
B Maldague	J Millon	C Montero	B Moyen
G de Mourgues	R Maigne	J P Moreau	P Poty
J O Ramadier	P Rochcongar	J Rodineau	J F Rabischond
A Ryckewaert	A Roux	G Saillant	P Sautre
S de Seze	A Trillat	J Vidal	F Viel
J Vittori	P Vancaver	F Vandervael	H Wagner

and others, for their help to the authors.

Chapter 1

INTRODUCTION

The knee is a highly modified hinge joint[1] that joins the femur to the tibia and to the patella. It is also a condylar unit[2] consisting of an overall structure that includes, from front to rear: the trochlea, which is the extension of the femoral condyles, and the patella, which is the extension of the tibial condyles (Figure 1.1).

However, the knee joint has two degrees of freedom:

The first degree, which involves flexion-extension movement of a 'true' hinge joint, acting similarly to the elbow.

The second degree, which involves rotary movement and is only possible in flexion. This can occur because this is both a 'modified' and 'incongruent' hinge joint.

It is 'modified' because its median crest, which includes the posterior median crest of the patella and the intercondylar eminence, is effectively incomplete.

It is 'incongruent' because its articular surfaces fit poorly into one another, in spite of the interposition of the menisci, which play the role of intercalary elements.

A complex, but solidly anchored and braced architecture is produced by a capsular, ligamentous and muscular system that is both powerful and highly perfected! This means that the knee can behave like a solid and inseparable functional unit, but that it is only as efficient as it is vulnerable, undoubtedly for the same reasons:

It is *efficient* in reconciling two *a priori* contradictory imperatives, *stability* (an indispensible condition for all joints of the lower limbs) and *mobility* (coexistence of two joints, the patellofemoral with one degree of freedom and the tibiofemoral with two degrees);

It is *vulnerable* because of the capsular and ligamentous components, which are frequently injured.

F. 1.1

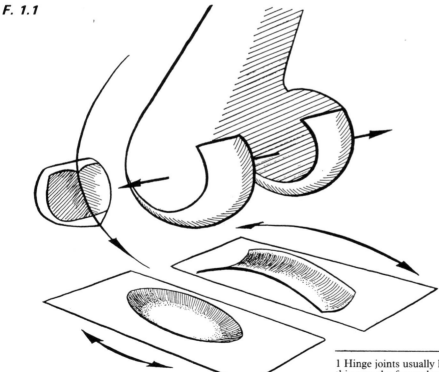

---

1 Hinge joints usually have one joint surface in the form of a pulley: in this case the femoral surface.

2 A condylar joint is a joint with cylindrical segments on the articular surface, one — in this case the femur — being convex, the other — in this case the patella and tibia — being concave.

Chapter 2
ANATOMY

The knee is described in its anatomical position of reference, in other words in extension.

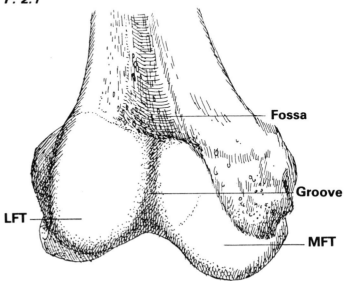

F. 2.1

Articular Surfaces[1]

The patellofemoral joint connects the femoral trochlea and the posterior facet of the patella.

The tibiofemoral joint connect the femoral condyles to the tibial condyles, though the menisci act as intermediaries to a great extent.

The proximal tibiofibial joint connects the facets of the corresponding heads of the tibia and the fibula.

Trochlea (Figures 2.1 and 2.2)

The trochlea is located on the anterior, distal end of the femur. There is an anteroposterior groove of the middle of the trochlea that divides it into two facets: the trochlear groove[2] opens on to the intercondylar notch to the rear; the lateral LFT and medial MFT facets are convex from all points of view. In a lateral view, they are similar to two spirals whose respective radii increase from front to rear. The two facets follow the condyles to the rear, going past the intertrochlear crests, with the lateral condyle being more clearly defined than the medial.

The general configuration has three distinct characteristics:

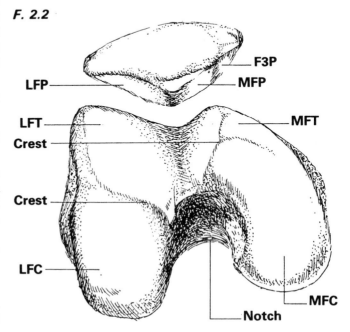

F. 2.2

- The lateral facet is further extended, more prominent and has a greater radius;

- The upper margin overhangs the supratrochlear fossa. There is a smooth transition between the fossa and the lateral facet, but a rougher transition to the medial facet;

- On the average, the angle of the trochlea T KK is 140°.

---

1 The cartiliginous covering and its thickness modify the traditional description.

2 The trochlear groove and the anatomical axis of the femur form an angle of several degrees, opening upward and outward.

Patella (Figures 2.2 and 2.3)

The patella is a sesamoid bone[3] integrated into the extensor apparatus between the quadriceps tendon QT and the patellar ligament PL (Figure 2.23).

There are three important characteristics that should be noted:

The thickness varies by a maximum of 2–3 cm, excluding the cartilage, while the cartilage may reach a thickness of 5 mm on the medial line[4].

The posterior facets consist of two parts, the superior articular and inferior extra-articular. The articular surface occupies the upper three-quarters and includes a crest and two facets: the prominent, blunt vertical crest corresponds to the trochlear groove; the two concave facets, lateral and medial, correspond to the trochlear facets; the lateral facet LFP is wider and not as oblique; the medial facet MFP integrates into the so-called third facet F3P of the tibial condyle, which only serves as a joint during extreme flexion.

The extra-articular point occupies the lower quarter of the patella and is partially occupied by the insertion of the patellar ligament.

● The average angle of the R KK is 130°.

F. 2.3

Femoral Condyles (Figures 2.3 and 2.4)

The condyles are located on the posterior, inferior part of the distal end of the femur. They are separated by the intercondylar notch and diverge toward the rear. The intercondylar notch is the continuation of the trochlear groove, while the lateral femoral condyle LFC and the medial condyle MFC make up the continuation of the corresponding trochlear facets. LFC and MFC are also convex from every point of view and therefore continue the two spirals, but their respective radii decrease from front to rear.

There are two essential characteristics that differentiate the lateral femoral condyle LFC from medial femoral condyle MFC:

● a larger surface area leading to a greater radius for the condylar spiral;

● less overall divergence toward the rear in relation to the sagittal plane, especially in the posterior third because it has a somewhat truncated shape[5].

F. 2.4

---

3 The resemblance to a sesame seed lies not only in the size and shape, but also on its location within the tendon, which lets it play the role of a reflection pulley.

4 The patellar cartilage is the thickest cartilage in the organism and is subject to the greatest pressure.

5 The anteroposterior axis is not straight, but can be regarded as having three parts: the anterior third slants to the rear and outward, the middle third is nearly sagittal and the posterior third oblique to the rear and inward. This means that divergence begins in the anterior third, is attenuated by the middle third and reversed by the posterior third.

Tibial Condyles (Figure 2.5)

The tibial condyles are located on the lateral and medial tuberosities[6] separated by the tibial intercondylar space: the lateral tibial condyle LTC and the medial tibial condyle MTC are transversely concave and articulate with the corresponding convex condyles. The tibial intercondylar space TICS narrows to the middle like an hourglass. The medial and lateral tubercules of the intercondylar prominence[7] are a reference point for the anterior and posterior intercondylar areas where the menisci and cruciate ligaments are attached.

There are major differences in terms of the sagittal curvature:

The lateral tibial condyle LTC is convex from front to rear starting at the top of the condyle TLTC, which is located at the junction of the anterior third and middle third: as a result, the surface is divided into two facets, an ascending anterior facet, and a descending posterior facet that forms a slight slope to join the posterior facet of the lateral tibial tuberosity.

The medial tibial condyle MTC is regularly concave from front to rear with a posterior margin of the medial tibial condyle PMT that overhangs the posterior surface of the medial tibial tuberosity.

On the whole, the convex medial femoral condyle and the concave medial tibial condyle fit into one another. On the other hand, the two convex surfaces of the lateral femoral and tibial condyles do not fit perfectly together (Figure 1.1).

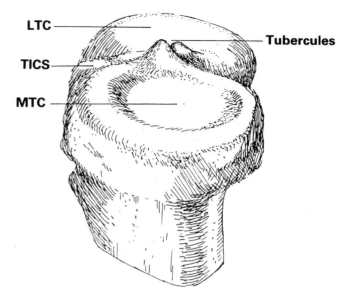

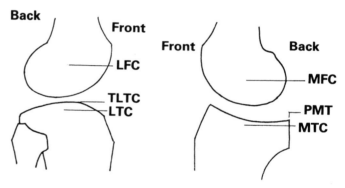

Proximal tibiofibular joint (Figure 2.6)

This is a plane joint[8] lying beneath the lateral tibial condyle at the level of the posterior third of the condyle.

The tibial surface occupies the posterior facet of the tibia's outer tuberosity. It is ovoid and faces backward, outward and downward.

The fibular surface occupies the medial facet of the head. It is also ovoid, but faces forward, inward and upward.

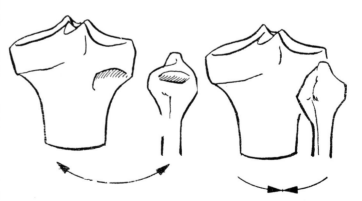

---

6 In profile the tibial plateau is not horizontal, but descends from front to rear.

7 The medial tibial tubercule MTT is higher and more anterior; its concave medial facet is an extension of the concavity of the medial tibial condyle MTC.

8 A plane joint has flat articular surfaces.

Synovial membrane (Figures 2.7 and 2.8)

From its point of attachment where the cartilage meets the bone, the synovial membrane Syn folds back on the bone, lining the rear surface of the capsule Cap and forming recesses or bursae of varying depth around the ends of the bones.

The perifemoral bursa is particularly evident in front of and opposite the supratrochlear groove, where it communicates with the subquadricipital serous bursa SQSB. The top of SQSB[9] is attached to the sub vastus intermedialis muscle (p. 24).

The peritibial bursa is mainly lateral and deeper toward the inside, sometimes several millimetres deep. The outside can communicate with the tibiofibular joint via a serous bursa lying beneath the popliteal tendon PT.

Since its sides are connected to the peripheral margin of the menisci (p. 15), the synovial membrane Syn can be regarded as having two sections, the meniscofemoral and the meniscotibial[10].

At the intercondylar notch, the rear of the synovial membrane Syn is invaginated as far as the fat pads (p. 22), passing around the two cruciate ligaments (p. 17). These ligaments are consequently extra-articular since they are extrasynovial, even though they are located within the capsule.

F. 2.8

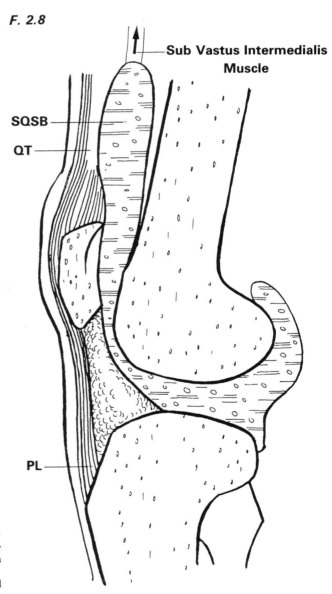

F. 2.7

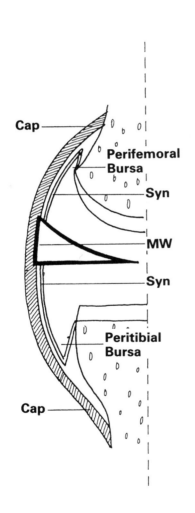

---

9 The subquadricipital serous bursa is occasionally separated totally or partially from the perifemoral pouch by a synovial fold that forms a closed area: the suprapatellar fold SPF.

10 The meniscus interrupts the synovial membrane but is not enveloped by it.

Means of attachment

The articular surfaces are attached to one another by a combination of menisci, ligamentous capsule, fat tissue and muscle.

Meniscal Apparatus (Figures 2.9–2.12)

The two menisci that are interposed between the tibiofemoral articular surfaces are of different shapes that nevertheless have the same general form and the same structural characteristics. The form varies in its dimensions but is proportional to the articular surfaces. It is easily recognizable by the following features:

The anteroposterior curvature terminates in anterior and posterior horns. These horns are attached to the anterior and posterior intercondylar areas respectively.

The triangular cross-section of a meniscus shows three surfaces and a border: the upper surface is concave from side to side and corresponds to the femoral condyle; the lower surface is nearly flat from side to side and corresponds to the tibial condyle. The thick, convex peripheral border forms the meniscal wall MW, which adheres to the capsule Cap, while the free, concave edge faces the intercondylar notch.

There are numerous attachments, some of which are highly individualized and constant:

- Intermeniscal by the transverse ligament TL, which is anterior to and extends between the anterior horns and is involved in the extensor apparatus (p. 23) through the infrapatellar fold IF (p. 22).

- Meniscotibial through the thick bundles of fibres that make up the fibrous horns of the menisci.

- Meniscocapsular through the attachments between the capsule Cap and the meniscal wall MW, which in front reinforce the lateral meniscopatellar ligament LMPL (p. 18) and the medial meniscopatellar ligament MMPL (p. 20).

The absence of a synovium characterizes these articular structures. They are the only 'non-synovialized' structures (p. 14).

The common structure is significant from both the macroscopic and microscopic points of view:

The macroscopic view consists of two zones:

- The peripheral zone covering a quarter of the meniscal area is called parameniscal because it is essentially vascular, starting at the capsule synovial level.

- The extended central zone covering three-quarters of the meniscal area is called articular because it is essentially fibrocartilaginous, and therefore capable of responding to articular requirements[11].

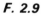

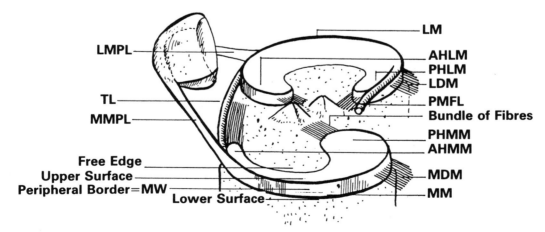

LMPL · TL · MMPL · Free Edge · Upper Surface · Peripheral Border=MW · Lower Surface · LM · AHLM · PHLM · LDM · PMFL · Bundle of Fibres · PHMM · AHMM · MDM · MM

---

11 The fibrocartilaginous structure is mixed, containing both tendon–capsule–ligament tissue and a cartilaginous covering.

On the basis of microscopic appearance, there are three groups of fibres:

- The most numerous are horizontal fibres that follow the anteroposterior curvature.
- Radial fibres predominate in the support zone, joining the peripheral surface and the free edge.
- Vertical or oblique fibres connect the upper and lower surfaces.

The lateral meniscus LM may have an eminently variable configuration, but among its most constant characteristics are:

- Its form is crescent-shaped, nearly a closed circle.
- The anterior horn AHLM is as large as the posterior horn PHLM.
- The peripheral surface attachment to the capsule is interrupted at the rear by the popliteal tendon PT, which crosses the posterior third at a more or less oblique angle through the popliteal hiatus PH.

Attachments are more numerous and reinforced. They consist of:

- Meniscofemoral, including the posterior meniscofemoral ligament PMFL that arises from the posterior horn and which is a satellite of the posterior cruciate ligament PCL[12].
- Meniscomuscular, including the lateral dynamic mooring LDM that connects the posterior horn PHLM to the popliteal tendon P (p. 5) and other structure (p. 30).

The medial meniscus MM has a particular but constant configuration:

- It is semilunar, nearly oblique.
- The slender anterior horn AHMM contrasts with the weight and thickness of the posterior horn PHMM.
- There is an uninterrupted attachment between the peripheral surface and the capsule.
- The attachments are reinforced with, among others, meniscomuscular attachments including the medial dynamic mooring MDM that connects the posterior horn PHMM to the straight head of the semimembranous muscle SM (p. 29) and associated structures.

---

12 The posterior meniscofemoral ligament crosses the PCL but more often anterior than posterior, sometimes splitting in two.

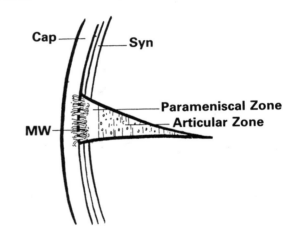

F. 2.10

Cap — Syn

Parameniscal Zone
Articular Zone

MW

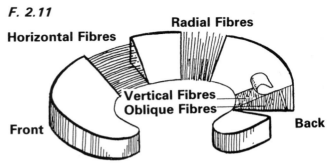

F. 2.11

Horizontal Fibres   Radial Fibres

Vertical Fibres
Oblique Fibres

Front   Back

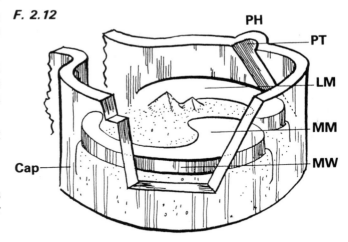

F. 2.12

PH
PT
LM
MM
MW
Cap

Capsular and ligamentous apparatus

The capsule and ligaments are made up of passive attachments combined in a central apparatus and a peripheral apparatus.

Central apparatus

The central apparatus consists of an essential *ligamentous part* and an accessory *osseous part*; consisting of the tibial spines.

Back

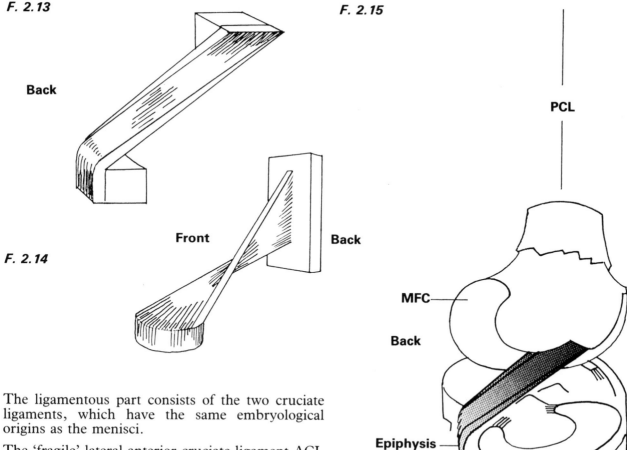

PCL

MFC

Back

Front   **Back**

Epiphysis

The ligamentous part consists of the two cruciate ligaments, which have the same embryological origins as the menisci.

The 'fragile' lateral anterior cruciate ligament ACL (Figures 2.13 and 2.14) has its anterior portion attached on the interior intercondylar area of the tibia near the anterior horn of the medial meniscus AHMM, just in front of the medial tibial tubercule MTT.

The lateral part is attached to the femur, vertical to and very posterior on the medial facet of the lateral femoral condyle LFC along a height that attains one-third of the length of the ligament. It extends obliquely upward, outward and to the rear. It is twisted so that the anterior fibres on the tibia become the medial fibres on the femur, normally in a multifascicular form[13]. Vascularization is uncertain[14].

The solid medial posterior cruciate ligament PCL (Figures 2.15 and 2.16) has its posterior part attached to the tibia, on the posterior intercondylar area at its most posterior section and continuing onto the tibial epiphysis. The medial part is attached to the femur, both horizontal to and extremely anterior on the lateral facet of the medial femoral condyle MFC, with a width that may attain the length of the ligament: It extends obliquely upward, inward and forward, and it is twisted so that the posterior fibres on the tibia become the lateral fibres

on the femur. Its large size is increased by the addition of other fibres, including those from the posterior meniscofemoral ligament PMFL (p. 16). Its vascularization is certain[15].

Synovial membrane

The synovial membrane encloses the two cruciate ligaments with a fold arising from the posterior facet of the joint (see above) and acting like a sleeve.

13 The multifascicular structure contains at least two bundles of fibres distinguished on the basis of how their tibial attachments are arranged: the long, slender anteromedial bundles of fibre and the short, thick posterolateral bundle.

14 The vascularization of ACL depends both on the middle articular artery and the periarticular arterial network via the fat pad (p. 22).

15 The vascularization of the PCL is largely provided by its attachment and by the medial geniculate artery.

F. 2.16

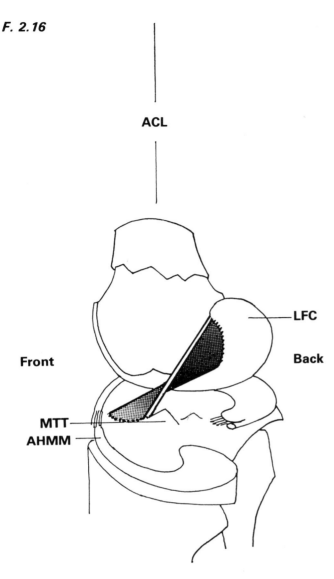

ACL

LFC

Front

Back

MTT

AHMM

Peripheral apparatus

The peripheral apparatus is the medial and lateral capsular and ligamentous unit, which will be outlined in three sections and separated into three levels; anterior, middle and posterior.

The three (usually highly unified) levels are:

● The deep capsular level which includes ligamentous reinforcements and thickenings.

● The middle, tendinous level.

● The superficial aponeurotic level, where the superficial aponeurosis is found in common with and in a continuity of the femoral aponeurosis from the top and the tibial aponeurosis from the bottom.

Lateral peripheral apparatus (Figure 2.17)

The anterior third is represented by the lateral patellar retinaculum LPR with the superimposition of:

> The capsule Cap adhering to the meniscal wall MW (p. 15) and reinforcing the lateral meniscopatellar ligament LMPL, which extends obliquely down, to the rear and the outside.

> The triangular lateral femoropatellar ligament LFL of the patella, extending from the base of the patella to the top of the lateral epicondyle of the femur, crossing behind the origin of the fibular collateral ligament (long) FCL-L.

> The vertical fibres of the vastus lateralis muscle and the horizontal fibres of the vastus medialis muscle (p. 24); fibres from the biceps and the tibialis anterior; the anterior fibres of the iliotibial band ITB, etc; the whole collection of fibres is always heterogeneous and discontinuous[16].

The middle third consists of the capsule, the iliotibial aponeurosis that doubles the front, and the fibular collateral ligament (long) that covers the rear.

> The iliotibial aponeurosis ITA has a posterior expansion (p. 27) that connects it to the lateral intermuscular septum LIMS (p. 23) of the thigh that arises on the lateral lip of the linea aspera of the femur.

> The fibular collateral ligament (long) FCL-L[17] starting at the long fibulofemoral fibres, bridging the lateral meniscus LM and the popliteal tendon PT to form a round cord-like ligament extending obliquely downward and to the rear.

> The proximal insertion is found on the lateral epicondyle of the femur LEF, just in front and crossed by the lateral femoropatellar ligament LFL.

> The distal insertion is on the lateral facet of the head of the fibula, enveloped by the biceps femoris tendon BT.

16 A zone of least resistance is formed by the two layer arrangement of a uniform superficial layer and a fasciculated lattice-type deep layer: the lateral front corner LFc corresponds to a recent description that is, nevertheless, difficult to confirm by dissection.

17 The fibular collateral ligament divides into a long and short ligament whose upper insertions are some distance from one another, but whose lower insertions approach to the point of merging. This produces the central V on the head of the fibula: the anterior and posterior branches, that respectively correspond to the long and short ligaments, are 'wrapped up' by the capsule, which divides into two layers at this point.

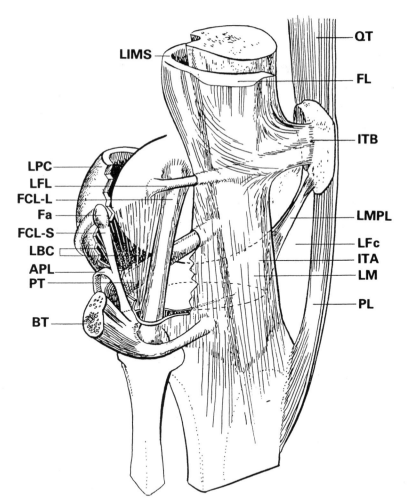

The posterior third is represented by the capsule as the basic element with increasing thickness from front to rear.

- The thick, strong posterior part covers the lateral condyle, forming the lateral posterior capsule LPC.

- The *proximal insertion* (Figure 2.29) combines with the insertion of the lateral head of the gastrocnemius LG, extending from the superior border of the lateral femoral condyle to the superior limit of the articular surface, sometimes even continuing onto the peripheral surface of the posterior horn of the lateral meniscus.

- The *distal insertion* is on the posterior facet of the lateral tibial tuberosity near the lateral tibial condyle.

The loose, thin anterior part forms the 'backdrop' of the zone of least resistance—the lateral back corner LBC. The LBC is like a window between the solid capsular, ligamentous and aponeurotic bands to the front and the thick lateral posterior capsule to the rear. It is not connected to the meniscus, but does have ligamentous support.

The separation between the LBC and the lateral meniscus is imposed by the lateral, oblique passage of the popliteal tendon PT: since the popliteal tendon is in contact with the peripheral surface of the meniscus, it interrupts capsular attachment along its length and this interruption is called the popliteal hiatus PH (Figure 2.12).

The ligamentous support of lateral back corner is provided by the fibular collateral ligament (short) FCL-S[17], which is a thick cord-like ligament extending obliquely downward and to the front.

- The upper insertion is on the fabella Fa.

- The lower insertion is on the apex of the head of the fibula, sharing the head with the insertion of the lateral band of the arcuate posterior ligament APL.

- The proximal tibiofibial joint is supported by ligaments, especially anterior and posterior, while still being able to communicate with the tibiofemoral joint.

Medial peripheral apparatus (Figure 2.18)

The anterior third consists of the medial patellar retinaculum MPR with the superposition of:

> The capsule Cap adhering to the meniscal wall MW (p. 15) and reinforcing the medial meniscopatellar ligament MMPL, which is less developed than its lateral counterpart, and extending obliquely downward, inward and to the rear.

> The medial femoropatellar ligament MFL is triangular in form; the base is attached to the patella, the top to the medial epicondyle of the femur and the rear to the tibial collateral ligament TCL, which it crosses at the level of the origin of the tibial collateral ligament.

> The vertical muscular expansions of the vastus medialis muscle and the transverse fibres of the vastus lateralis muscle (see below), and other structures, produce a rather uniform and continuous unit in relation to the lateral anterior third (p. 18).

The middle third combines the middle capsule and the tibial collateral ligament that covers it.

The middle capsule is made up of short fibres terminating in the meniscus, making it possible to distinguish the meniscofemoral fibre bundle from the meniscotibial bundle.

The tibial collateral ligament TCL is very well distinguished, starting from the long tibiofemoral fibres, bridging the medial meniscus and the horizontal groove below the medial tibial condyle, where the reflected head of the semimembranous muscle RfT SM is positioned. The tibial collateral ligament therefore forms a strong band because it is broad, thick, and extended obliquely downward and to the front. The oval-shaped upper insertion is on the medial epicondyle of the femur and just in front of the insertion of the medial femoropatellar ligament MFL which it crosses; the thin and widespread lower insertion is on the anterosuperior part of the medial surface of the tibia, extending downward and to the rear of the insertion of the muscles of the pes anserinus PA and the interposed anserine bursa.

The posterior third is represented by the capsule as the basic element, with increasing thickness from front to rear.

The thick, strong posterior part covers the medial femoral condyle forming the medial posterior capsule MPC. The upper insertion (Figure 2.29) is on the upper border of the medial femoral condyle and is closely linked to the insertion of the medial head of the gastrocnemius MG, whereas the separation between capsule and muscle most often starts immediately, creating a cleavage plane that can be transformed into a medial gastrocnemius bursa MGB and which can communicate with the joint. The lower insertion is on the posterior surface of the medial tibial tuberosity, several millimetres below the posterior margin of the medial tibial condyle.

The thin, loose anterior part forms the 'backdrop' of the zone of least resistance: the medial back corner MBC.

Like a 'window' between strong capsular and ligamentous bands in front and the thick medial posterior capsule to the rear, the MBC has meniscal and musculoligamentous support. The medial meniscus MM supports the MBC by peripheral attachment to the capsule (Figures 2.10 and 2.12).

Musculoligamentous support of MBC is provided by the semimembranous muscle SM and the posterior oblique ligament POL. The semi-membranous muscle SM makes up the medial dynamic mooring MDM (p. 16) and participates in delimiting the MBC with its three tendons (p. 30): reflected head RfT, straight head StT and recurrent head RcT. Starting at its posterior femoral insertion on the adductor tubercle, the posterior oblique ligament POL diverges obliquely through the MBC with its three fibre bundles: upper F up, middle F mid and lower F low.

On the whole, MBC support is 'tentacular' in form with the interweaving of three tendons and three fibre bundles: in fact, the upper bundle follows the recurrent head, the middle bundle integrates into the straight head and the lower bundle passes over the reflected head before terminating behind the tibial collateral ligament on the tibia.

Fat apparatus

The fat apparatus consists of the fat pad and its expansions arising from the synovial membrane (Figure 2.19).

The infrapatellar fat pad FP is a fatty mass that fills the cavity limited to the front by the point of the patella and the patellar ligament PL, and below by the anterior intercondylar area of the tibia.

The fatty and cellular expansions make up the alar fold and the infrapatellar fold: the alar folds are lateral rolls of fat that extend along the lower half of the borders of the patella, and the infrapatellar fold

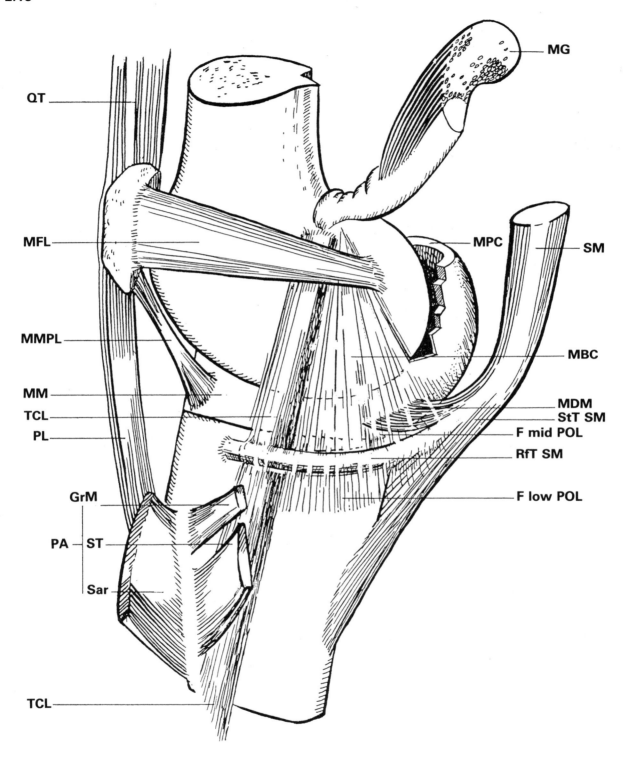

QT

MG

MFL

MPC

SM

MMPL

MM

TCL

PL

MBC

MDM

StT SM

F mid POL

RfT SM

GrM

PA — ST

Sar

F low POL

TCL

IF is posterior, a cord-like structure that arises from the middle of the fat pad and finds its insertion on the end of the intercondylar notch, sometimes extending up to the anterior cruciate ligament ACL (p. 17), following an intra-articular path, obliquely backward and upward in the sagittal plan[18].

The synovial membrane covers this largely fatty fold, separating it from the joint cavity[19].

The pretibial bursa PTB is located below the fat pad, between the proximal end of the tibia and the patellar ligament PL.

F. 2.19

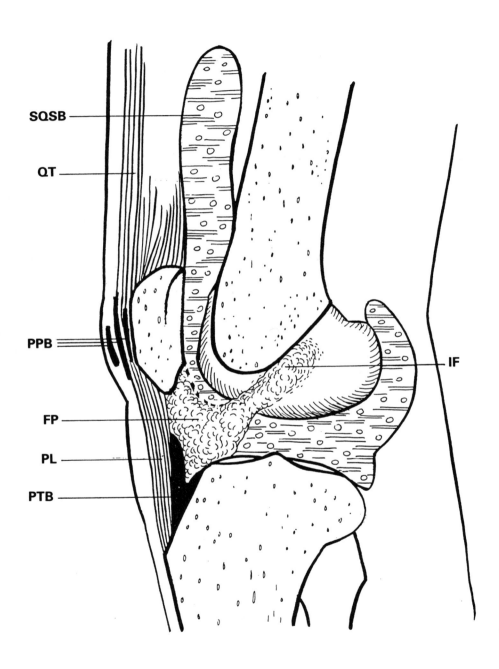

SQSB

QT

PPB

FP

PL

PTB

IF

---

18 This is the vestige of a median septum that continues up the sagittal septum in the fetus, and is subsequently reduced to a suspensory ligament.

19 The synovial membrane that covers the fat pad, is sometimes attached to the medial surface of the medial trochleocondylar junction by a synovial fold that forms a band extending obliquely backwards from the patella, the retropatellar fold RPF.

Muscle and tendon apparatus

This is the active 'harness' that is broken down into four muscle groups, plus the popliteal muscle, which is considered separately.

1. Anterosuperior group

The quadriceps occupies practically the whole anterior compartment of the thigh (Figure 2.20). It is innervated by the femoral nerve[20], and is the predominant element in the extensor apparatus.

The origins of the quadriceps enable us to break it down into four heads:

a) Rectus femoris RF (Figures 2.20, 2.21 and 2.22).
The superficial head is the only muscle of the quadriceps that crosses two joints (hip and knee). The tendon sheath of origin combines the straight head StT from the anterior inferior iliac spine and the reflected head RfT from the rear of the rim of the acetabulum, which forms its pathway, and the recurrent head RcT from the anterosuperior angle of the greater trochanter. The tendon sheath then descends quite low, remaining superficial to the body of this muscle.

b and c) Vastus lateralis muscle VL and vastus medialis muscle VM (Figures 2.22–2.25).
These lateral heads give rise to two muscles that cross a single joint (knee). Their origin is in the aponeurotic sheath that spreads over the entire linea aspera: the vastus lateralis muscle is attached to the lateral surface in front of the lateral intermuscular septum LIMS and continues up to the greater trochanter; the vastus medialis muscle is attached to the medial lip in front of the medial intermuscular septum MIMS and continues up to the lesser trochanter.

The vastus medialis muscle is distinguished on approaching the knee by an extensive deployment of fibres. To the extent that we can separate them into contingents, the superior contingent follows the shaft of the femur forming the longitudinal part of the vastus medialis VML; the inferior contingent slants obliquely forming the oblique part of the vastus medialis VMO[21], which fuses with the lower fibres of the adductor magnus muscle deep in the leg, and serves the particular function of providing support to the front of the medial femoropatellar ligament MFL (p. 20) and the medial border of the patellar ligament PL through its aponeurotic band.

---

20 Terminal branch of the lumbar plexus.
21 The distinction between VML and VMO is essentially physiological in nature.

F. 2.20

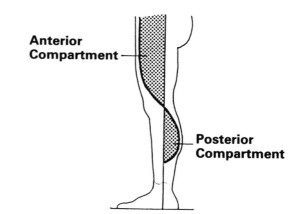

F. 2.21

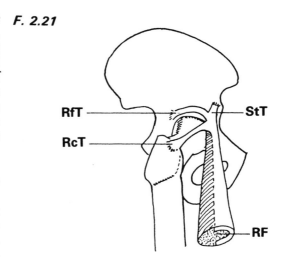

F. 2.22

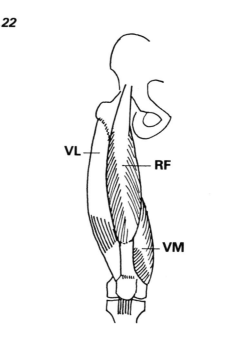

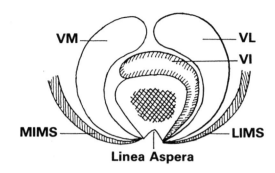

F. 2.23

VM — — VL

— VI

MIMS — — LIMS

Linea Aspera

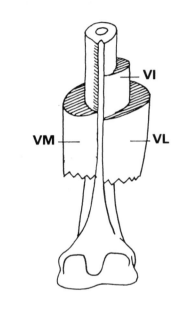

F. 2.24

— VI

VM — — VL

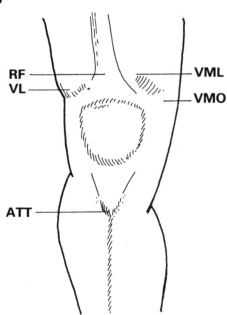

F. 2.25

RF —
VL — — VML

— VMO

ATT —

d) Vastus intermedius VI (Figures 2.23 and 2.24).
The deep head is moulded around the convex part of the femur. This muscle crosses a single joint (knee). The straight head cloaks the anterior and lateral surfaces of the femur. It is close to the origin of the vastus lateralis muscle and is separated from that of the vastus medialis muscle by the medial surface of the femur, which is free of any attachment. The Sub vastus intermedius provides deep attachment for the subquadricipital bursa SQSB (p. 14) on the anterior surface of the femur. It terminates by merging with the quadriceps tendon, which is an expansion of the patellar ligament which reinforces aponeurotic expansions and serous bursae, all of which combine to make up a tendinous and aponeurotic parallelogram:

Quadriceps tendon QT (Figures 2.26 and 2.27) (also Figures 2.17–2.19).
The QT consists of four terminal tendons that merge several centimetres above the patella and subsequently join the base of the patella. There are three levels:

The tendon of the rectus femoris RF occupies the superficial level, rising high on the leg and eventually plunging deeply to the fleshy fibres of the muscle; however, a distal expansion extends over the patella to make up the superficial part of the patellar ligament.

The tendons of the vastus lateralis muscle VL and the vastus medialis muscle VM merge in the middle level upon arriving from the deep and superficial facets of their respective muscles; however, the terminal tendon of the oblique part of the vastus medialis VMO opens toward the bottom, extending its insertion onto the upper superior, medial border of the patella.

The tendon of the vastus intermedius VI occupies the deepest level, rising very high on the leg and becoming superficial where it meets the fleshy fibres of its muscle.

Patellar ligament PL (Figures 2.27 and 2.28) (also Figures 2.17–2.19)
This is a broad, flat ligament that diminishes in size from top to bottom. The upper insertion consists of a wide attachment on the point of the patella; the lower insertion is on the anterior tibial tuberosity[22], whereas the superior part of the lower insertion is separated by the pretibial bursa PTB (p. 22).

22 The proximal head of the tibia consists of three projections: the anterior tibial tuberosity ATT, a triangular area on the lower head which is found between the lateral tibial tuberosity and medial tibial tuberosity, which are located on either side of the head.

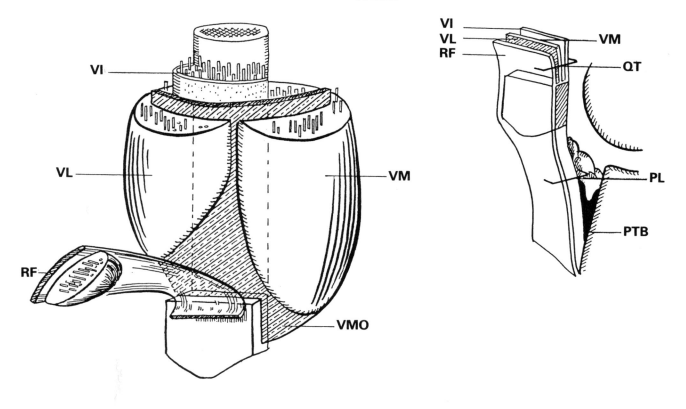

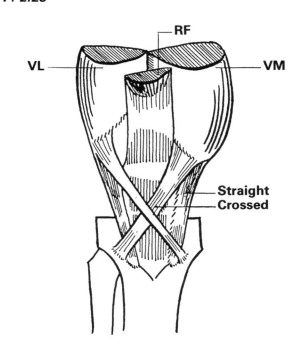

The tendinous and aponeurotic expansions (Figure 2.28)

These expansions consist of a double anterior reinforcement.

Higher and deeper on the leg, the straight and crossed expansions of the terminal tendons of the vastus lateralis muscle and vastus medialis muscle are arranged symmetrically but with clear medial dominance.

The direct longitudinal expansion is attached to the lateral border of the patella and the patellar ligament, and to the corresponding tibial tuberosity.

The crossed expansion passes over the median line, in front of the patella and the patellar ligament and is attached to the opposite tibial tuberosity.

At the bottom, on a superficial level, the common expansion of the fascia lata and the sartorius muscle lies against the anterior face of the patellar ligament (pp. 27 and 29).

The prepatellar bursae PPB are called subcutaneous, middle and deep. They are superimposed even though they are inserted between tendinous and aponeurotic levels (Figure 2.19).

2. Posteroinferior group (Figures 2.29–2.31)

The lateral head of the gastrocnemius LG and the medial head of the gastrocnemius MG are directly involved in knee movement: they are the two superficial heads of the triceps surae[23] of femoral origin. This is a muscle that crosses more than one joint (knee and rear of foot). It is integrated into the posterior compartment of the leg (Figure 2.20) and is innervated by the medial popliteal nerve[24].

The upper origin is symmetrical, both posteriorly and posterolaterally (Figures 2.29–2.30):

The posterior origin is straight, with upper fibres inserted on the epicondyles and lower fibres merging with the posterior capsule. However, the height at which the muscle merges with the posterior capsule varies in relation to the joint space: the common insertion of the lateral head of the gastrocnemius LG and the lateral posterior capsule LPC descends very low (p. 19), reaching the level of the posterior horn of the lateral meniscus and even exchanging fibres with its peripheral surface; on the other hand, the separation of the medial head of the gastrocnemius MG and the medial posterior capsule MPC occurs at a high common insertion, creating a plane of cleavage that forms the medial gastrocnemius bursa MGB (p. 20).

The posterolateral origin is indirect, starting from a tendon inserted laterally on the epicondyle just above the upper insertion of the tibial collateral ligament: the tendon of the lateral head of the gastrocnemius LG is subtended by the fabella Fa[25] whereas the tendon of the medial head of the gastrocnemius MG extends its insertion below and behind the tubercule of the adductor magnus AM, the two tendons of origin descend very low while fanning out superficially where they connect with their fleshy fibres.

However, the crossing between the tendon of origin of the medial head of the gastrocnemius and the reflected head of the semimembranous muscle

(p. 30) takes place through tight, direct overlapping: this results in a crimp that can be opened to provide communication between the gastrocnemio-semimembranous bursa GSB of the medial head of the gastrocnemius and the semimembranous muscle with the medial gastrocnemius bursa MGB, which is connected directly to the joint (p. 20).

The lower part terminates on the common tendon that appears in the middle of the leg: by extending very far upward, the common tendon separates around the two heads of the gastrocnemius and remains deep in relation to the belly of the muscle; in descending, the common tendon joins the terminal tendon of the soleus, thereby forming the Achilles tendon.

F. 2.29

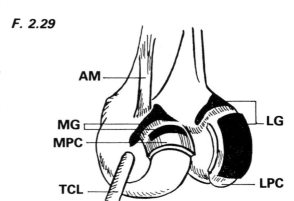

F. 2.30

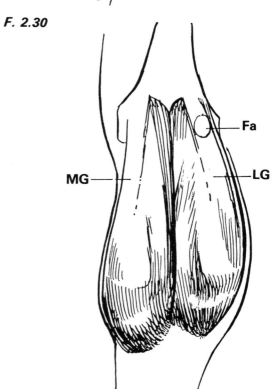

---

23 The soleus is the deep head of tibal origin.

24 Terminal branch of the greater sciatic nerve.

25 The fabella, Latin for 'little bean', is interposed between the tendon of the lateral gastrocnemius and the lateral posterior capsule. Initially fibrous, then cartilaginous and finally osseous, the fabella is, in fact, a true sesamoid whose more highly elaborated contours show two surfaces: the concave and cartilaginous anterior surface is integrated into the capsule. The constancy of the fabella, which is at least represented by a thickening of the capsule, makes it a 'corner stone' toward which structures converge and insert, since by necessity certain parts merge though their origins are different: the fibular collateral ligament (short) (p. 19), the oblique popliteal ligament (p. 30), the arcuate popliteal ligament through an expansion of the lateral pillar (p. 31).

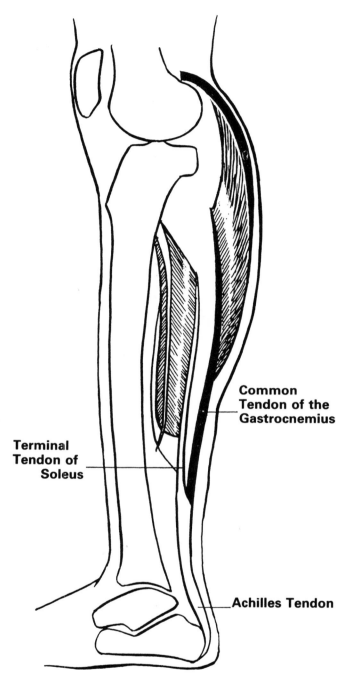

Common Tendon of the Gastrocnemius

Terminal Tendon of Soleus

Achilles Tendon

a) Fascia lata FL (Figure 2.32)

The upper origin of the fascia lata merges with the gluteus muscles GlM. It originates in a broad semiconical attachment, mainly on the iliac crest, and is innervated by the superior gluteal nerve[26]. The lower end terminates in a thick, strong and consequently so-called 'solid' tendon that covers the whole upper, lateral surface of the thigh. It is to a great extent inserted into the anterolateral surface of the tibia[27], linked to the femoral and then tibial aponeurosis, with a double and practically indistinguishable tibiofemoral expansion.

● The iliotibial aponeurosis ITA consists of both the terminal tendons of the fascia lata, the gluteus maximus and gluteus aponeurosis, combining in a posterior expansion at the lateral intermuscular septum of the thigh LIMS (Figure 2.17).

The iliotibial band ITB reinforces the lateral patellar retinaculum (p. 18) with two anterior expansions, one superior and horizontal that is inserted into the lateral border of the patella (Figure 2.17), the other lower and arc-like expansion wraps around the patellar ligament, coming together in an expansion similar to the sartorius muscle (Figure 2.35).

On the whole, the fascia lata and the sartorius muscle (p. 29) merge at their upper insertion on the anterior superior iliac tubercule, forming two thin strips of a frond that hems in the patellar ligament leaving an anterior concave depression.

b) Biceps B (Figures 2.32–2.33)

The upper origin links the biceps to the ischiotibial muscles in a common plane with the semitendinous ST and posterior to the semimembranous muscle SM. Arising on the ischium, integrated into the posterior compartment of the thigh and innervated by the sciatic nerve, the long head of biceps doubles in size at the mid thigh and outside of the short head of the biceps SB, which is inserted on the lateral lip of the linea aspera.

The lower end terminates in a thick tendon that merges with the two portions on the lateral facet of the head of the fibula, enclosing the lower insertion of the fibular collateral ligament (long) FCL-L with the interposition of a serous bursa and continued by anterior tibial expansions.

3. Posterolateral group

This is a small group consisting of the fascia lata and the biceps, which pass over two joints (hip and knee).

26 Collateral branch of the sacral plexus.

27 It is inserted on the tubercule of the anterior surface of the lateral tibial tuberosity and on the crest that links the lateral to the anterior tibial tuberosity.

F. 2.32

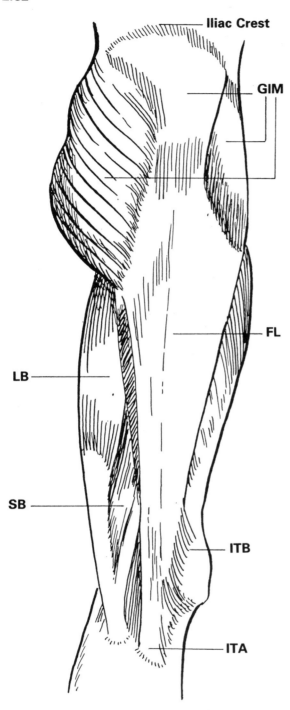

- Iliac Crest
- GIM
- FL
- LB
- SB
- ITB
- ITA

F. 2.33

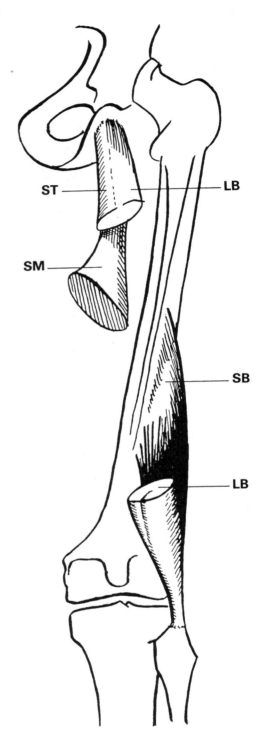

- ST
- LB
- SM
- SB
- LB

4. Posteromedial group

This group consists of four muscles that cross two joints (hip and knee): the semimembranous muscle is the 'head of the group', fanning out behind the three pes anserinus muscles.

a) (The pes anserinus PA muscles (Figures 2.34–2.35) The tibial termination is the single commonpoint of these muscles, and consists of the three tendons that slide over the medial surface of the proximal tibia, where a serous bursa separates them from the tibial collateral ligament.

The differentiation is based on the origin[18], topography, innervation and morphology:

Sartorius muscle Sar: arising on the anterior superior iliac tubercule ASIT, and integrated into the anterior compartment of the thigh[29], the sartorius muscle slants[30] across the anteromedial surface of the thigh like a ribbon under the femoral aponeurosis and joins an expansion of the fascia lata FL (p. 27). It is supplied by the femoral nerve.

Gracilis muscle GrM: arising from the pubis, the gracilis is integrated into the medial compartment of the thigh[31]. The gracilis is vertical and establishes the medial limit of the thigh. It is innervated by the obturator nerve[30].

Semitendinous muscle ST: arising on the ischium, the semitendinous muscle is integrated into the posterior compartment of the thigh[32], is innervated by the sciatic nerve[33], is already tendinous at the mid thigh and is attached by an expansion of the aponeurosis of the medial gastrocnemius MG.

The junction occurs on the proximal part of the medial surface of the tibia (Figure 2.18), just behind the tibial crest[34] and in front of the lower insertion of the tibial collateral ligament TCL, on two levels that are indistinguishable in appearance. In front and throughout the upper part, the sartorius muscle Sar tendon fans out, sending an expansion outward toward the fascia lata (p. 27) and forward toward the tibial aponeurosis. To the rear, the gracilis muscle GrM tendon and the semitendinous muscle ST are superimposed from top to bottom.

F. 2.34

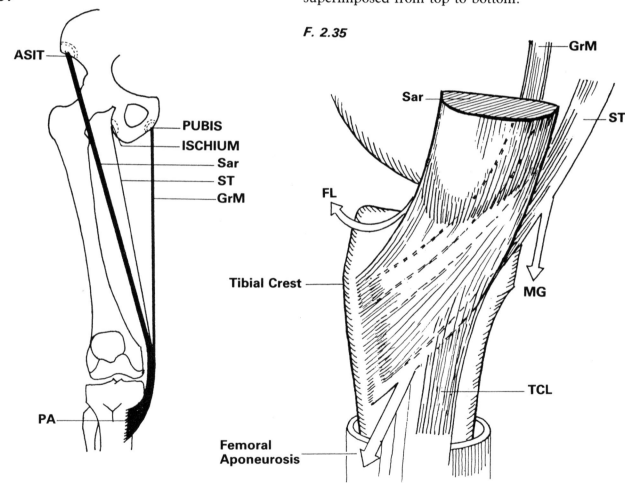

F. 2.35

---

28 The origin is based on the three points of insertion that are the highest on the ilium, showing that, among the thigh muscles, the sartorius is the most anterior, the gracilis muscle is the most medial and the semitendinous is the most posterior.

29 The anterior area is almost completely occupied by the quadriceps, which is deep to the other muscles.

30 Terminal branches of the lumbar plexus.

31 The adductor area.

32 The hamstring area.

33 Terminal branch of the sacral plexus.

34 Anterior border of the tibia.

b) Semimembranous muscle SM (Figure 2.36)

The upper origin links the semimembranous muscle to the ischiotibial muscles, but anterior to the semitendinous muscle ST and the long head of the biceps LB: arising on the ischium, the semi-membranous muscle is integrated into the posterior compartment of the thigh. It is distinguished by its thin descending tendon which arrives at mid thigh before enlarging. It is innervated by the greater sciatic nerve.

The lower end terminates in an insertion complex of three tendons facing the posterior medial angle of the tibia (Figure 2.37).

The straight head StT continues the direction of the muscle when the knee is extended, and inserts on the posterior facet of the medial tibial tuberosity (Figure 2.18): the straight head is integrated into the MBC (p. 20) and is connected to the posterior horn of the medial meniscus PHMM forming the medial dynamic mooring MDM (Figures 2.9 and 2.18).

The reflected head RfT continues the direction of the muscle when the knee is flexed at a right angle. It follows the lateral transverse groove below the medial tibial condyle, passing under the tibial collateral ligament TCL and is inserted into the anterior surface of the medial tibial tuberosity (Figure 2.18): the reflected head is integrated into the MBC and is involved in the communication of the posterior serous bursae.

The recurrent head RcT slants upward and outward in the popliteal fossa, merging with the lateral posterior capsule LPC and inserting mostly on the fabella Fa (p. 26 and note 25), forming the oblique popliteal ligament OPL: the reflected head is integrated into the MBC (p. 20) and is connected to the popliteal muscle through an expansion.

Popliteal muscle P (Figure 2.37)

All aspects of this seemingly isolated muscle distinguish it from other muscles[35].

- This is the only muscle crossing a single joint (knee) that is both extra-articular (fleshy fibres) and intra-articular (tendon), and is located deep within the popliteal fossa.

- The particular morphology of a short, flat, triangular muscle: the tibial base corresponds to the fleshy body which is inserted on the

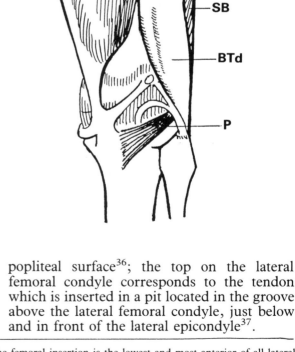

popliteal surface[36]; the top on the lateral femoral condyle corresponds to the tendon which is inserted in a pit located in the groove above the lateral femoral condyle, just below and in front of the lateral epicondyle[37].

---

35 Up to the present time the popliteal muscle was not very well understood and not extensively studied.

36 The upper third of the posterior tibial facet.

37 The femoral insertion is the lowest and most anterior of all lateral femoral condyle insertions.

38 Intra-articular communication through the tendon benefits from a passage between the capsule and the synovium or an underlying serous bursa linked to the lateral peritibial pouch (p. 13).

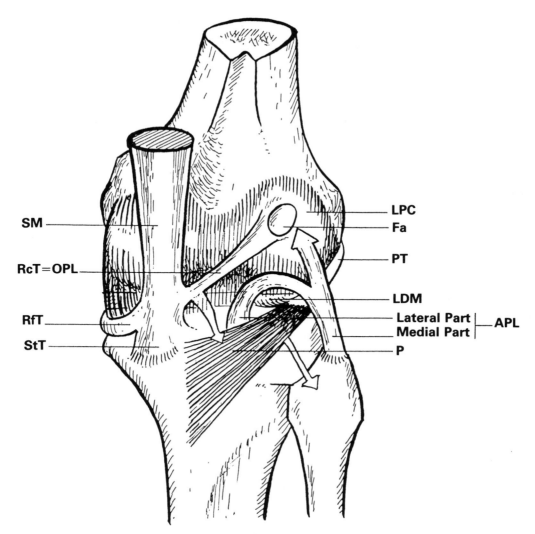

SM

RcT=OPL

RfT

StT

LPC
Fa
PT
LDM
Lateral Part | APL
Medial Part |
P

● The unusual orientation upward, outward and forward, in a favourable position to encircling because it is nearly horizontal (Figure 2.17).

● It is supplied by the medial popliteal nerve.

Its intimate relationships are:

Above, the intra-articular tendon, which makes for easier communication between the tibiofemoral and the proximal tibiofibial joints[38].

Outside, the intra-articular tendon slants across the LBC and the fibular collateral ligament (short) FCL-S, then the fibular collateral ligament (long) FCL-L (Figure 2.17).

Inside, the intra-articular tendon slants across the peripheral surface of the lateral meniscus, interrupting the attachment to the capsule and forming the popliteal hiatus PH (Figure 2.12).

Below, the fleshy extra-articular part is integrated into the posterior compartment of the leg.

In front, the flesh-tendon junction is located at the edge of the posterior border of the lateral tibial condyle. It is connected to the posterior horn of the lateral meniscus PHLM, forming the lateral dynamic mooring LDM (Figure 2.9); (p. 15).

To the rear, the flesh-tendon junction merges with numerous connections of the popliteal fossa: the semimembranous muscle through an expansion of the oblique popliteal ligament OPL, which is inserted into the lateral posterior capsule LPC and the fabella Fa; the posterior cruciate ligament PCL, the arcuate posterior ligament APL, whose low, concave ligamentous arch bridges between the lateral[39] and the medial[40] parts of the APL; head of the fibula, and neighbouring structures.

---

39 The lateral pillar is located on the apex of the head of the fibula and with an expansion resting on the fabella (p. 26 and note 25).

40 The medial part rests on both the lateral posterior capsule and the tibia just above the base of insertion for the fleshy part of the popliteal muscle.

Chapter 3
BIOMECHANICS AND KINETICS[1]

The knee is subject to a large number of demands that are essentially brought about by muscular contraction. However, weight-bearing may enter into the picture[2] in an accessory sense, through inertia and occasionally through outside manoeuvres[3], but these result in torque[4] of mobility-stability forces[5], both intermittently and with two particular features.

Torque only occurs in flexion, which creates movement[6]; extension is the counterbalance, resulting in immobility.

Torque occurs in an active–passive manner, theoretically being split into two components:

- *Passive mobility*—passive stability torque represents passive torque through the voluntary participation of articular surfaces and of the meniscal, capsular and ligamentous system, which is constantly under tension.
- *Active mobility*—active stability torque represents active torque through voluntary participation of the muscular system and weight-bearing.

In order to understand the biomechanics and consequent practical applications, we will analyse the knee even further by using a theoretical basis of reference:

Breaking down this unified and inseparable functional unit into its various components will enable us to analyse the behaviour of the passive knee and then the active knee, first in extension, then in flexion, with separate analyses of the patellofemoral and tibiofemoral joints.

The theoretical reference point is the tibia, whether the leg is free in a lying position or fixed in a standing position.

Passive knee

Voluntary participation of articular surfaces and the meniscal, capsular and ligamentous system[7] differs depending on whether the knee is extended or flexed:

Extension terminates in immobility, with two significant features: only the tibiofemoral joint participates, and passive torque is balanced out, producing passive stability[2].

Flexion makes movement possible, with two significant features: participation of the patellofemoral joint with a single degree of freedom and the tibiofemoral joint with two degrees of freedom; and the passive torque comes into play in order to establish a compromise between passive mobility and passive stability[8].

Weight-bearing can always be balanced by the single passive knee: the articular surfaces and the meniscal, capsular and ligamentous system are consequently capable of controlling the tendency of the centre of gravity to shift outside the foot support area.

F. 3.1

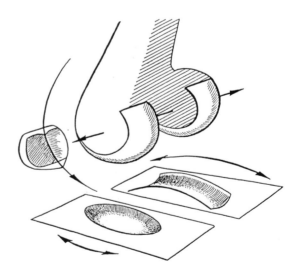

---

1 The study of the biomechanics and kinetics of movement is based essentially on theoretical deductions.

2 Weight-bearing, in other words gravity, body weight, etc., is visualized in terms of the centre of gravity of the whole body; this centre of gravity is located in front of the lumbosacral joint and is vertical to the balance-maintaining and support surface of the feet (**Note:** the support surface or base of support corresponds to the area within the outside edges of the feet, tangent to the tips of the toes and the heels).

3 The manoeuvres are used in tests for abnormal movements, etc.

4 The torque of forces is a concept used in mechanics to describe twisting, i.e. parallel and equal but opposite forces.

5 Stability to some extent corrects or compensates for mobility; knee movement can therefore be monitored, blocked, suppressed, slowed, balanced or contained, as desired.

6 The concept of torque of forces applies to movement analysed into moments or phases.

7 A lesion of the meniscal, capsular and ligamentous system is the key feature in an injury that is considered either as serious because of tearing disinsertion, or as benign because of distension.

8 Decrease or loss of passive stability resulting from a lesion of the meniscal, capsular and ligamentous system leaves abnormal mobility and consequently abnormal movement that signifies a serious sprain.

'Passive Knee' in extension

Only the tibiofemoral joint contributes to immobility through passive stability (p. 32).

The patellofemoral joint (Figures 3.2 and 3.3)

The patellofemoral joint does not participate in extension, during which time the patella is in its high position. At this point the patella is prominently visible within the extensor apparatus; it is disaligned and capable of transverse movement:

Having nearly entirely left the trochlea, the patella moves into the supratrochlear fossa[9] and slightly outward[10] in its high position.

Integrated into the extensor apparatus, the patella can be identified by its centre C[11] which is located at the junction of the axis Q of the quadriceps tendon and the axis R of the patellar ligament, the latter being inseparable from the anterior tibial tuberosity ATT.

- In the frontal plane, C is located within Q and R, the slant of Q being due to the orientation of the trochlear groove (p. 11 and Note 3, p. 12) and the orientation of R to the lateral position of ATT: this means that the extensor apparatus is disaligned, forming an angle QCR of YY 170° but becoming wider when the patella is shifted outside of the supratrochlear fossa[10].

- In the sagittal plane, C is located in front of Q and R, the slant of Q being due to the essentially posterior origin of the quadriceps and R due to the posterior location of ATT: this means that the extensor apparatus is non-aligned, forming an angle QCR of 1YY 165°.

F. 3.3

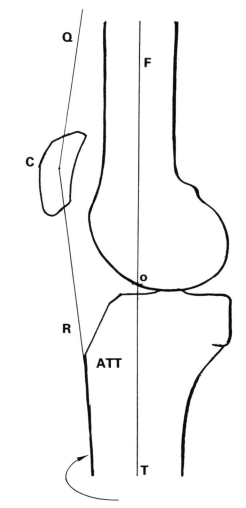

$$Q\hat{C}R = 165°$$
$$F\hat{O}T = 180°$$

F. 3.2

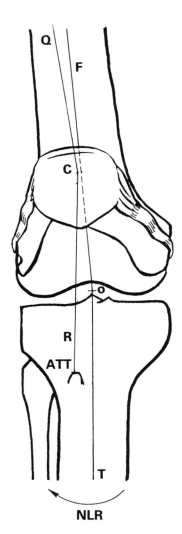

$$Q\hat{C}R = 170°$$
$$F\hat{O}T = 174°$$
$$L\hat{R}T = 5°$$

NLR

---

9 The patellar cartilage has lost contact with the trochlear cartilage and is now in contact with the synovial fold of the subquadricipital pouch.

10 The lateral position of the patella may create a pitfall in looking for the bayonette sign.

11 The centre C of the patella corresponds to its functional centre.

Being freed of the trochlea, the patella can move transversely, nearly equal distances to either side, with the lateral femoropatellar ligament (p. 18) and medial femoropatellar ligament (p. 20) controlling, respectively, medial and lateral movement.

Tibiofemoral joint (Figures 3.2 and 3.3)

This is the only joint involved in extension, while stability is acquired passively by frontal disalignment and lateral alignment of the anatomical axes[12] along with lateral rotation of the tibia.

In the frontal plane (Figure 3.2), the disalignment of the anatomical axes of the femur F and of the tibia T form physiological valgus, with the angle FOT of YY 174° equalling physiological genu valgum.

In the sagittal plane (Figure 3.3), the alignment of the anatomical axes of the femur F and the tibia T corresponds to a vertical line that serves as the reference for 0° of extension, but with the possibility of physiological genu recurvatum equal to YY −10°.

In the horizontal plane[13] (Figure 3.2), the tibia is immobilized under the femur in LRT of YY 5° representing the final point of necessary lateral rotation during the transition from flexion to extension (p. 40).

On the whole the 'passive' knee can attain submaximum stability, with passive control accomplished by locking the knee in the extended position (Figure 3.4).

Passive control calls into play the whole capsular and ligamentous system:

● Passive control uses all elements that form the central apparatus even though the ACL and the PCL are uncrossed and a maximum distance apart, in fact nearly parallel in the sagittal plane (Figure 3.5): the lateral femoral condyle LFC is 'anchored' by the ACL which is in a 'standing' position (Figure 3.7) ready for shortening[14]; at the same time, the medial femoral condyle MFC is 'retained' by the PCL which is in a 'lying down' position (Figure 3.7) that is suitable for stretching[15].

12 The anatomical axis corresponds to the diaphysial axis, which is both median and longitudinal for the femur F and the tibia T.

13 The horizontal plane in the standing subject becomes vertical in the subject who is lying down.

14 In relation to its tibial insertion, the femoral insertion of the anterior cruciate ligament is both closest and highest in extension: closest, in that the ACL is called upon to stretch, thereby using its lengthening possibilities; highest in that the ACL is 'vertical' or 'standing up'.

15 In relation to its tibial insertion, the femoral insertion of the PCL is both furthest and lowest in extension: furthest in that the PCL is called on to stretch; lowest in that the PCL is 'horizontal' or 'lying down'.

F. 3.4

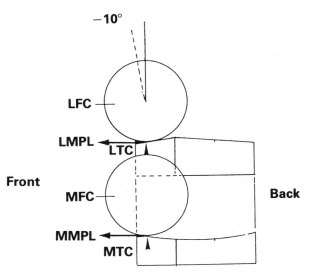

F. 3.5

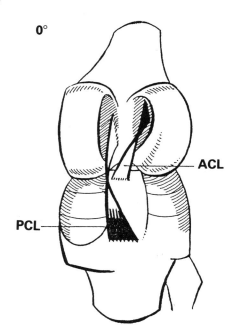

F. 3.6

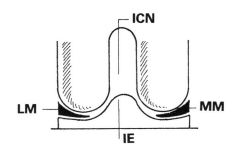

34

F. 3.7

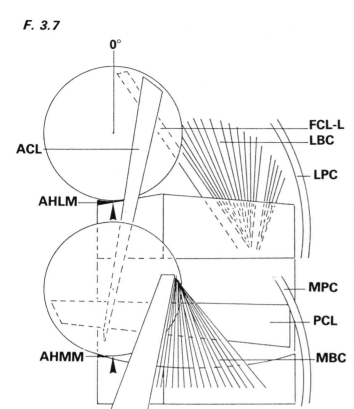

0°

ACL

FCL-L
LBC

LPC

AHLM

MPC

PCL

AHMM
MBC

TCL

● Passive control uses all elements that make up the medial and lateral apparatus.

The extended position is attained when the lower limb is straight, in other words with the leg stretched to the maximum, but passively, at the hip. Locking is assured by congruency, and capsular and ligamentous resistance.

The congruency of the articular surfaces is attained in the frontal plane (Figure 3.6), facilitated by the way that the convex femoral condyles fit into the concave tibial condyles[16], consolidated in the centre by a 'key' made up of the intercondylar eminence IE and around the periphery by the adjustment of the menisci LM and MM[17] which are pulled forward by the meniscopatellar ligaments LMPL and MMPL (Figure 2.9). Capsular and ligamentous resistance is perfect or nearly so (Figure 3.7).

Lateral security is obtained by stretching of the posterior cruciate ligament PCL in the centre[15], by the fibular collateral ligament (long) FCL-L and the lateral back corner LBC for outward movement, and by the tibial collateral ligament TCL and the medial back corner MBC for inward movement. All of which makes it impossible for any lateral opening of the tibiofemoral space to occur[18].

To the rear, the thick strong lateral posterior capsule LPC and medial posterior capsule MPC reinforce the 'solid' posterior cruciate ligament PCL like a 'safety lock'.

To the front, security is always compromised because it relies on a single ligament, the anterior cruciate ACL, which is only called upon to stretch to its maximum in recurvatum.

The 'passive knee' during flexion

The patellofemoral and the tibiofemoral joints are involved in movement that makes use of passive torque.

The patellofemoral joint

Only one degree of freedom is involved in this joint, and the 'passive' mechanism is therefore simple.

The basic sequence of movements results from a combination of mobility/stability operations.

Passive mobility occurs essentially at the trochlea, where movement results from sliding[19], while the patella remains equidistant from the tibia (Figure 3.8). The trochlea slides progressively upward and backward, the patella being held in place at ATT by the inextensible patellar ligament PL.

Passive stability mainly occurs at the patella, with lateral support provided by the patellar retinacula and the lateral facet of the trochlea (Figure 3.9).

The patellar retinacula LPR and MPR are first called into play (pp. 18 and 20), making use of their possibility of stretching as flexion continues[20]. This stretching is particularly marked in the medial retinaculum[21].

---

16 The femoral condyles are always more convex than the tibial condyles are concave.

17 The adaptation of the menisci in extention makes perfect adjustment of the osseous elements possible, particularly in terms of the femoral condyles whose convex surfaces can entirely correspond to the concave superior facets of the menisci: the largest support zone is consequently reached in extension, because of the larger radii of curvature of the femoral condyles (p. 12) and the interpositions of the menisci.

18 The valgus VI extension E Test = VIE; varus Vr extension E Test = VrE; drawer D extension E = DE; the big B toe T = BT.

19 The patellofemoral joint combines the conditions necessary for sliding that would double friction: the friction that occurs in sliding becomes very forceful when resistance is offered by a patella in direct contact with the trochlea.

20 Since flexion involves progressing along a trochlear spiral whose radii of curvature increase (p. 11), the patellofemoral ligaments stretch to a greater extent as their insertions become further and further apart.

21 The medial patellar retinaculum MPR is called upon to stretch to the maximum because of its growing obliqueness in the direction of the medial epicondyle (p. 12).

F. 3.8

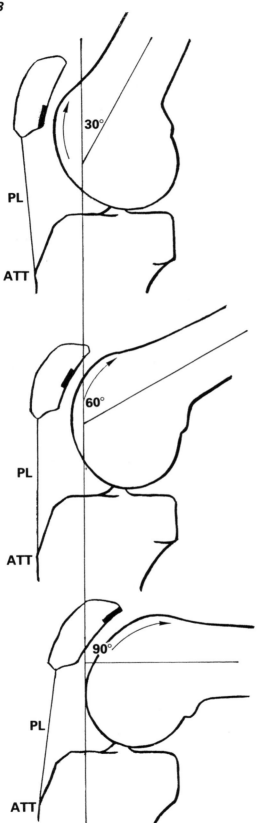

The lateral facet of the trochlea LFT is larger and more prominent, and blocks lateral movement of the patella once it has entered the groove, i.e. once flexion has begun.

F. 3.9

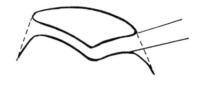

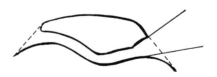

Sequential biomechanics at 30°, 60° and 90° essentially show gradual changes in the behaviour of the patella.

In the frontal plane, the patella has to recentre itself in order to take a more medial position, tip over and respond to the alignment of the extensor apparatus:

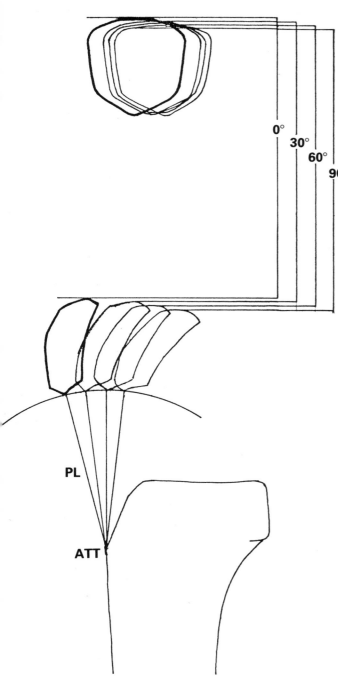

F. 3.10

0°
30°
60°
90°

PL

ATT

In responding to the alignment of the extensor apparatus, the patella enables the angle QCR to open and become a straight line (Figures 3.19, 3.28, 3.29, 3.36 and 3.37).

In the sagittal plane, the patella changes support and moves rearward:

In approaching the trochlea (Figure 3.8), the patella only partially presents its articular surface[22]: the lower third at around 30°, the middle third at around 60°; the upper third at around 90°, the lateral borders and articular facets of the third facet of the patella (p. 11) beyond 90°.

In moving rearward with the femur (Figure 3.9), the patella follows the arc of a circle that is centred on the anterior tibial tuberosity ATT with a radius equal to the length of the patellar ligament PL[23] to situate itself in relation to the ATT: in front at 30°, direcly vertical at 60° and to the rear at 90°, which has the effect of attenuating the narrowing in the angle QCR at 30°, 60° and 90° (Figures 3.20, 3.28, 3.29, 3.36 and 3.37).

The tibiofemoral joint

The tibiofemoral joint has two degrees of freedom and a complex passive interaction.

The basic biomechanics involve a combination of mobility/stability operations that work through a central regulatory mechanism and the adjustment of the menisci. The combined mobility/stability operations imply the existence of relative mobility and relative stability.

Passive mobility occurs basically in the lateral compartment and as the result of the lateral femoral condyle having an appropriate shape.

- The extensive surface of the lateral femoral condyle (p. 12) provides it with a large capacity for development.

- The least divergence toward the rear of the lateral femoral condyle makes demands on the lateral capsule and ligaments by shortening them, and consequently opening the possibilities of stretching.

Upon leaving the supratrochlear fossa, the patella positions itself at the entry to the trochlear groove and appears to plunge in while being subjected to various recentering oscillations around a relatively fixed position (Figure 3.8).

In tipping over, the patella opens the medial patellofemoral interline whose edges diverge inwards (Figure 3.9).

---

22 The support varies but at the cost of reducing the articular surfaces of the patella to one-third of its total area, which has the effect of multiplying unitary pressure three times!!! At the same time, if the patellar cartilage, the thickest cartilage in the organism, is capable of resisting high pressures, the lower and middle thirds are 'fragile': in fact, this is the support zone that is called into play most often and the one that is in greatest danger, particularly in athletes, in spite of its limited participation in the abnormal demands arising from an imbalance in the extensor apparatus.

23 The patellar ligament PL is incapable of stretching.

● The two opposing convex surfaces, the lateral femoral and tibial condyles do not really fit into one another.

Passive stability basically occurs in the medial compartment and as a result of the medial femoral condyle having the appropriate shape, for similar but opposite reasons.

F. 3.11

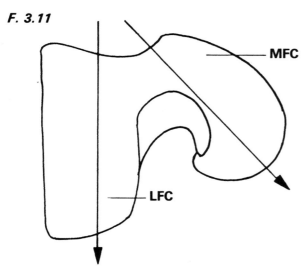

F. 3.12

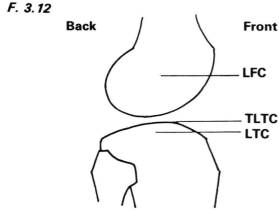

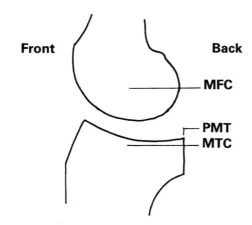

● The reduced surface of the medial condyle provides it with a limited possibility of development.

● Extensive divergence toward the rear of the medial femoral condyle makes demands on the medial capsule and ligaments at close to maximum stretching.

● The two opposing convex medial femoral and concave medial tibial condyles fit into one another very well.

The regulatory mechanism acts at the centre of the tibiofemoral joint, in other words in the intercalary compartment, through so-called necessary rotation.

The *intercalary compartment* corresponds to the tibial intercondylar space TICS in the intercondylar notch ICN and is where bone is joined to ligament.

The bone is accessory: it consists of the intercondylar eminence IE, which already participates in transverse blocking and more particularly in extension (Figure 3.6).

The ligament is essential: this is the central apparatus (p. 16), in other words the two cruciate ligaments that anchor the two femoral condyles provide control and, in the same respect, verify the rolling QQ sliding of the two condyles[24].

In extension ZZ flexion, the rearward movement of the femur proceeds from rolling ZZ sliding of both femoral condyles[25]. The lateral femoral condyle LFC is immobilized at the beginning, because it is 'anchored' in extension by the shortening of the 'standing' anterior cruciate ligament (Figure 3.7). The LFC frees itself as soon as flexion is initiated, first rolling, then sliding (Figure 3.13): rolling Rl only occurs in the first 25° of flexion, benefiting from the relative mobility of the lateral compartment and the possibility of lengthening the 'lying down' anterior cruciate ligament ACL; the

---

24 The combination of the rolling that occurs in the meniscofemoral articulation and the sliding that occurs in the meniscotibial articulation provide two basic advantages:

● an increase in the range of joint movement while maintaining articular relationships: in fact flexion would soon arrive at its limit, both in isolated rolling (Figure 3.15) that would terminate in posterior dislocation of the femoral condyle, as well as in isolated sliding (Figure 3.16) that would result in the femoral diaphysis jamming against the posterior tibial border.

● reduction of friction on articular surfaces: in fact, friction occurring during sliding and the minor friction of rolling are absorbed by the menisci providing an enormous advantage to the tibiofibular joint as opposed to the patellofemoral joint (p. 35 and Note 21).

25 The rolling-sliding combination corresponds to a series of events: pure rolling Rl initiates flexion, with sliding progressively taking over from rolling Rl + Sl. As flexion increases, pure sliding Sl occurs at the end of flexion.

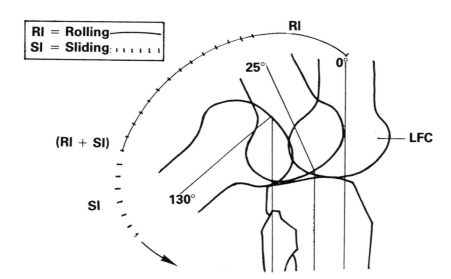

| RI = Rolling ———— |
| SI = Sliding: ı ı ı ı ı ı |

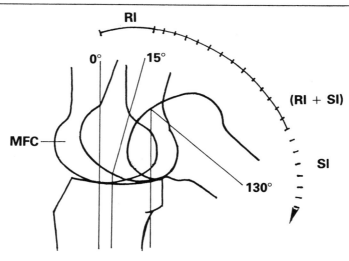

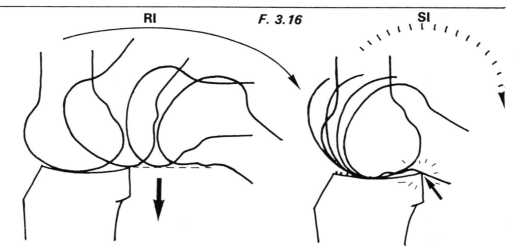

sliding Sl manifests itself secondarily as soon as the lateral femoral condyle LFC is retained in the flexed position by the lengthening of the 'lying down' anterior cruciate ligament ACL (Figure 3.32).

The MFC is immobilized at the beginning because it is retained in extension by the lengthening of the PCL, which 'lies down' (Figure 3.7). It frees itself simultaneously as soon as flexion is initiated, but in order to roll less and slide more (Figure 3.14): only rolling Rl occurs in the first 15° of flexion, being limited by the relatively stationary medial compartment and by the impossibility of further stretching the posterior cruciate ligament PCL which 'stands up'. On the other hand, sliding is anticipated as soon as the medial femoral condyle MFC is 'anchored' in flexion by the shortening of the 'standing' PCL (Figure 3.33).

In flexion ZZ extension, the forward movement of the femur reproduces the movement of the femoral condyles in the opposite direction, sliding ZZ rolling[26].

Necessary rotation is based on the condylar spirals of the femur (p. 12) whose asymmetry[27] makes it possible to develop the necessary medial rotation NMR in flexion and necessary lateral rotation NLR in extension.

In extension ZZ flexion, the necessary medial rotation NMR enables the anterior cruciate ligament ACL and the posterior cruciate ligament PCL to cross one another, and the extensor apparatus to align itself.

- The two cruciate ligaments touch each other at their axial borders and cross one another[28], producing a coadaptation that is well suited to stability (Figure 3.17).

- The extensor apparatus progressively aligns itself with the tibial-femoral axis in the frontal plane (pp. 34–37–41–45), resulting in a decrease in lateral demand, and creating a situation appropriate to stability.

- On the whole, the destabilization that begins with the initiation of flexion is somewhat corrected by a double stabilizing effect that takes place in the so-called 'stable' medial compartment (p. 37).

In flexion ZZ extension, necessary lateral rotation NLR enables the anterior cruciate ligament ACL and the posterior cruciate ligament PCL to uncross, and the extensor apparatus to disalign itself.

- The two cruciate ligaments uncross and no longer maintain any contact[29], producing a decoadaptation that is well-suited to mobility (Figure 3.18).

F. 3.17

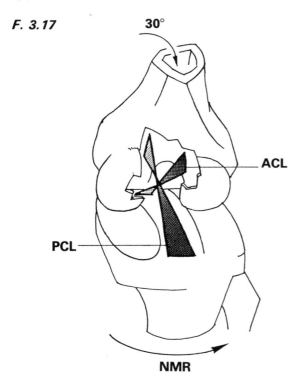

NMR

F. 3.18

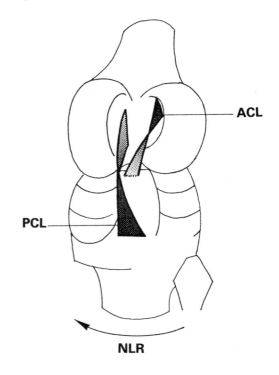

NLR

---

26 The sliding-rolling combination corresponds to the opposite series of events: pure sliding Sl at the end of flexion, the sliding being gradually overtaken by rolling Sl + Rl, whereas when flexion is decreasing, pure rolling Rl occurs at the approach to extension.

27 Equivalent to an automobile differential gear.

28 The ACL makes good use of its stretching potential (p. 34 and Note 14) to twist around the PCL.

29 The ACL is once again able to stretch (p. 34 and Note 14), moving sufficiently far from the PCL to become parallel to it.

- The extensor apparatus progressively loses its alignment with the tibiofemoral axis in the frontal plane, resulting in an increase in lateral demand and creating a situation appropriate to mobility.

- On the whole, the stabilization, which begins as soon as extension is approached, is somewhat corrected by the double destabilizing effect occurring in the so-called 'mobile' lateral compartment (p. 38).

The adjustment of the menisci to the articular interaction takes place within the limits of the intermeniscal, meniscotibial and meniscocapsular attachments: through deformation[30], the menisci can subsequently follow the femoral condyles[31] but to the detriment of articular congruity[32].

Sequential biomechanics

Sequential biomechanics at 30°, 60° and 90° of flexion combines frontal alignment, lateral disalignment and free rotation of the tibia under the femur.

In *30° of flexion*, in relation to extension (p. 33):

In the frontal plane, alignment begins to occur (Figure 3.19):

- alignment of the anatomical axes of the femur and the tibia eliminate the angle FOT of physiological valgus;

- the alignment of the extensor apparatus, made necessary by a medial shift of the anterior tibial tuberosity in order to accomplish necessary medial rotation of the tibia (p. 41), widens the angle QCR.

F. 3.19

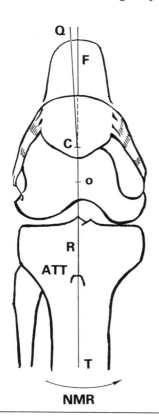

QĈR = 177°
FÔT = 180°

NMR

F. 3.20

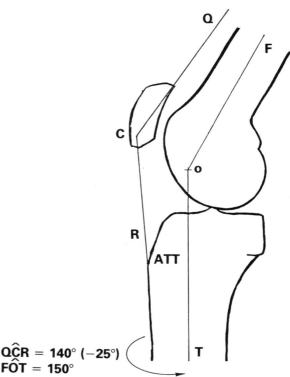

QĈR = 140° (−25°)
FÔT = 150°

30 Deformation affects the general contour of the menisci, but does not affect the cross-sectional view (p. 15). This can occur because the menisci have a fibrocartilaginous structure that provides them with both resistance and elasticity.

31 The course of the lateral meniscus, with its intimate links to the conditions existing in the lateral compartment (p. 38) is twice as long as that of the medial meniscus.

32 The adaptation of the menisci in flexion is the opposite of the effect produced in extension (p. 35 and Note 17), and does not offer the possibility of adapting precisely to bone, even though the cross-section cannot be deformed: the support zone decreases to nearly one-half of its surface in complete flexion, but less than one would expect from the decrease in the radii of curvature of the femoral condyles (p. 12), because of the interposition of the menisci.

In the sagittal plane, disalignment increases (Figure 3.20):

- alignment of the anatomical axes of the femur and the tibia forms the angle of flexion;

- disalignment of the extensor apparatus increases, narrowing the angle QCR, but less than would be indicated for the angle of flexion, because of the rearward movement of the femur-patella (p. 37).

In the horizontal plane, free rotation of the tibia under the femur acquires a certain amplitude because of additional mobility controlled by the peripheral stabilizers. This range of rotation averages 30°, largely relying on the 'mobile' lateral compartment (p. 37). The axis of rotation is near the medial compartment[33] and moves backwards with flexion[34].

Additional sagittal mobility (p. 38) occurs in relation to a reference position defined as the zero point in free rotation[35]. In rotation O RO, simultaneous rolling-sliding of the femoral condyles[36] occurs from front to rear, leading to a new position

F. 3.21

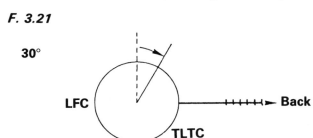

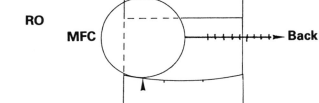

F. 3.22

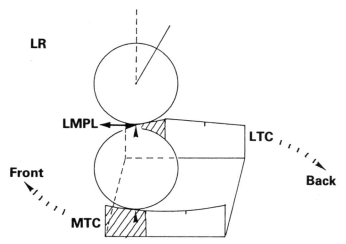

F. 3.23

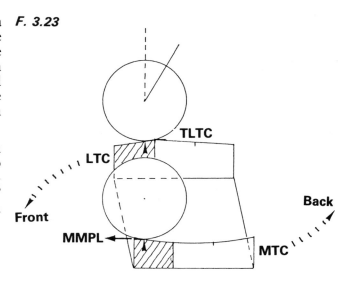

of the articular surfaces, in which the middle of the respective anterior thirds of each surface meet (Figure 3.21). In free lateral rotation LR or medial rotation MR dual tibial condyle sliding[37] takes place alternately and in the opposite direction, making it possible to sweep over the largest stretch of the articular surfaces, covering the respective anterior thirds and even going beyond (Figures 3.22 and 3.23).

In lateral rotation LR (Figure 3.22):

● Rearward sliding of the lateral tibial condyle LTC enables the lateral femoral condyle LFC to descend onto the anterior facet of the tibial condyle, returning to the position it initially held in extension (Figure 3.4), a process assisted by the lateral meniscopatellar ligament LMPL (p. 15) which maintains the lateral meniscus LM in a forward position;

● Forward sliding of medial tibial condyle MTC enables the medial femoral condyle MFC to continue its descent toward the bottom of the concave part of the tibial condyle.

---

33 The axis of rotation is close to the medial tibial tubercule in extension.

34 The axis of rotation moves backwards with flexion, following the arc of an expanding circle outside of the medial compartment.

35 The reference position is determined by the foot, with the big toe pointed toward the ceiling.

36 The rolling-sliding of the two femoral condyles at 30° of flexion takes over from pure condylar rolling that occurs at the beginning of flexion (p. 38 and Note 25).

37 There is no rotation in tibial condyle sliding.

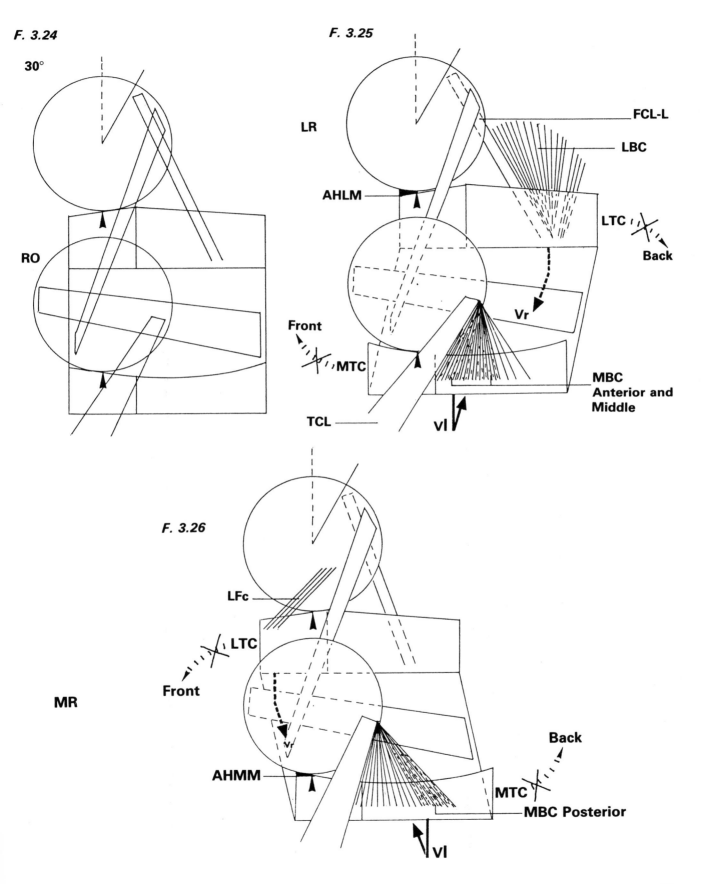

F. 3.24

30°

RO

F. 3.25

LR

FCL-L

LBC

AHLM

LTC

Back

Front

MTC

Vr

TCL

vl

MBC
Anterior and
Middle

F. 3.26

MR

LFc

LTC

Front

Vr

AHMM

Back

MTC

MBC Posterior

vl

In medial rotation MR (Figures 3.24 and 3.25):

- forward sliding of the lateral tibial condyle LTC enables the lateral femoral condyle LFC to conclude its ascent on the anterior facet of the tibial condyle, but without being able to reach the top of the lateral tibial condyle TLTC, which marks the limit between the anterior and middle thirds (p. 13).

- the forward sliding of the medial tibial condyle MTC enables the medial femoral condyle MFC to return to the position it originally held in extension (Figure 3.4), benefiting from the assistance of the medial meniscopatellar ligament MMPL (p. 15), which retains the medial meniscus MM in a forward position.

- When stretched, the lateral peripheral stabilizers are subject to demands that counteract any lateral opening in the tibiofemoral space.

In lateral rotation LR (Figure 3.25):

- Abduction or valgus Vl is controlled[38] by the tibial collateral ligament TCL and the anterior and middle parts of the medial back corner MBC (p. 20).

- Adduction or varus Vr is controlled[39] by the fibular collateral ligament (long) FCL-L and the lateral back corner LBC.

In medial rotation MR (Figure 3.26):

- abduction or valgus Vl is controlled[40] by the posterior part of the medial back corner MBC.

- adduction or varus Vr is controlled[41] by the lateral front corner LFc (p. 18 and Note 16) beyond the lateral physiological opening permitted by the fibular collateral ligament (long) FCL-L[42].

F. 3.27

60°

Q F

C

O

R

ATT

QĈR = 180°
FÔT = 180°

T

NMR

F. 3.28

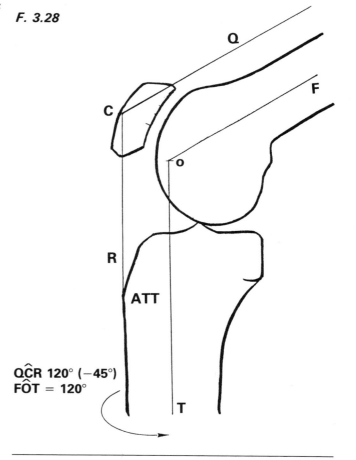

Q

F

C

O

R

ATT

QĈR 120° (−45°)
FÔT = 120°

T

---

38 Valgus Vl lateral rotation LR Test = VlLR.
39 Varus Vr lateral rotation LR Test = VrLR.
40 Valgus Vl medial rotation MR Test = VlMR.
41 Varus Vr medial rotation MR Test = VrMR.

42 The movement to the rear by lateral femoral condyle LFC and lateral tibial condyle LTC to the front, brings the insertions of the fibular collateral ligament (long) (p. 18) closer together and diminishes its initial slant downward and backward: this enables the fibular collateral ligament (long) FCL-L to 'rise' and thereby shorten its length, subsequently offering possibilities of stretching that create a small lateral physiological opening, VrMR = +.

In *60° flexion* in relation to 30° flexion (p. 41):

In the frontal plane, complete alignment is obtained (Figure 3.27):

- The angle FOT of physiological valgus has become a straight line.
- The angle QCR has become a straight line.

In the sagittal plane, disalignment increases (Figure 3.20).

- The angle of flexion has doubled.
- The angle QCR narrows, but less than would be anticipated by the angle of flexion, the correction due to the femur–patella moving rearward so that the ATT is subsequently located directly under the patella.[43]

In the horizontal plane, the greatest free rotation of the tibia under the femur is due to additional mobility controlled by stabilizers that are both peripheral and central. On the average a maximum range of movement of 40° is reached, with the axis of rotation even in further to the rear and closer to the posterior cruciate ligament PCL.

The additional sagittal mobility takes place in relation to a reference position defined as the zero point in free rotation (p. 42 and Note 35).

- in rotation O RO (Figure 3.29), simultaneous rolling-sliding of the femoral condyles[44] occurs from front to rear, leading to a new position of the articular surfaces in which the middles of the respective middle thirds of each surface meet. In lateral rotation LR or medial rotation MR dual tibial sliding[45] takes place alternately and in opposite directions, sweeping across the largest stretches of the articular surfaces.

In lateral rotation LR (Figure 3.30):

The rearward sliding of the lateral tibial condyle LTC enables the lateral femoral condyle LFC and the lateral meniscus LM to return to their initial extension position (Figure 3.4): the condyle once again crosses the top of the lateral tibial condyle TLTC, going down the facet of the anterior tibial condyle, until blocked by the anterior horn of the lateral meniscus AHLM[46] which is held in a forward position by the lateral meniscopatellar ligament LMPL (pp. 15 and 18).

The rearward sliding of the lateral tibial condyle LTC enables the medial femoral condyle MFC and the medial meniscus MM to become situated in relation to their respective posterior thirds: the condyle advances up the posterior facet of the concave surface of the tibial condyle until it is blocked by the voluminous posterior horn of the medial meniscus PHMM[47], which is pulled rearward by the medial dynamic mooring MDM (pp. 16 and 30).

F. 3.29

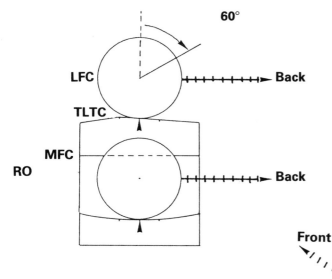

F. 3.30

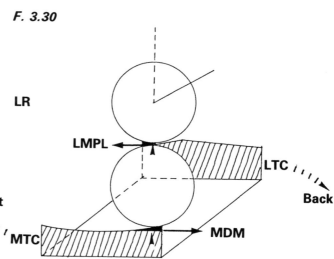

---

43 At 60° the points of reference C-R-ATT are aligned on the same vertical line, but only if the tibia itself is vertical.

44 At 60°, both femoral condyles roll and slide, pure sliding only taking place at the end of flexion (p. 38 and note 25).

45 There is no rolling in tibial condyle sliding.

46 The PHLM finally stops the lateral tibial condyle LTC from escaping to the rear.

47 The posterior horn of the medial meniscus PHMM finally prevents the medial tibial condyle MTC from escaping forward and the medial femoral condyle MFC from slipping out to the rear (Figure 3.30).

In medial rotation MR (Figure 3.31):

The forward sliding of the lateral tibial condyle enables the lateral femoral condyle LFC and the lateral meniscus LM to situate themselves in relation to their respective posterior thirds: the femoral condyle concludes its descent of the posterior facet of the tibial condyle until it is blocked by the posterior horn of the lateral meniscus PHLM[48], which is pulled rearward by the lateral dynamic mooring LDM (pp. 16 and 31).

The rearward sliding of the medial tibial condyle MTC enables (in principle) the medial femoral condyle MFC and the medial meniscus MM to return to their initial extension positions (Figure 3.4): the femoral condyle ascends the anterior facet of the concave part of the tibial condyle while the MM is retained forward by the medial meniscopatellar ligament MMPL (pp. 15 and 20), an effort always limited, undoubtedly the result of being wedged in[49].

During stretching, demands are made on the rotary central and peripheral stabilizers (pp. 17–19–20) to counteract any subluxation of the tibia.

In rotation O RO, forward QQ rearward stability is under complete control (Figure 3.32).

The advance of the tibia from the tibial intercondylar space TICS[50] is held in check by a two-part system: (1) The first part of this system consists of the anterior cruciate ligament ACL, which comes into play beyond the limits of acceptable physiological drawer sign[51]. (2) The second part consists of the medial back corner MBC, which is sufficiently 'well-armed' with support from the meniscus, muscles and ligaments (p. 20) to assist the relatively fragile anterior cruciate ligament ACL and possibly to back up that assistance with the aid of the lateral front corner LFc (p. 18 and Note 16).

The rearward movement of the tibia from the tibial intercondylar space TICS[52] is substantially controlled by the 'solid' posterior cruciate ligament PCL (p. 17).

F. 3.31

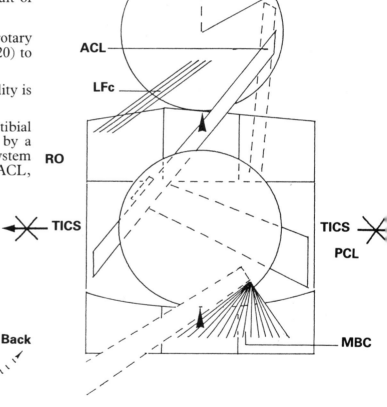

F. 3.32

---

48 The posterior horn of the lateral meniscus PHLM finally prevents the lateral tibial condyle LTC from escaping forward and the lateral femoral condyle LFC from slipping out to the rear (Figure 3.32).

49 The medial femoral condyle MFC skids as soon as it is clear of the medial tibial condyle MTC, while the propensity for being wedged in can be explained as follows: the reciprocal fit (p. 38), the double stabilizing effect of the necessary medial rotation (p. 40), the absence of anterior dynamic recall, etc. Being as slender as it is (p. 16), the anterior horn of the medial meniscus AHMM does not participate in blocking continued movement.

50 The voluntary V anterior A drawer D sign = VAD and the anterior drawer AD rotation O RO = ADRO.

51 The anterior cruciate ligament ACL has stretching possibilities (p. 40 and Note 28) which can produce a limited physiological drawer sign, ADRO = +.

52 The voluntary V posterior P drawer D = VPD and the posterior P drawer D rotation O RO = PDRO.

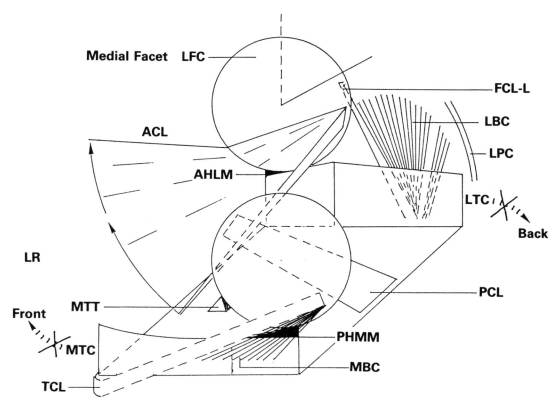

In the lateral or medial free rotation, rotary stability takes the form of a highly perfected gradual control in lateral rotation, but a rather summary control in medial rotation.

In lateral rotation LR, control is highly perfected (Figure 3.33); the forward movement of the tibia from medial tibial condyle MTC[53] is subject to an extremely 'geared down' 'braking system'.

(1) The 'main brake' is provided by the combined action of the medial back corner MBC and the posterior horn of the medial meniscus PHMM. The medial back corner MBC responds immediately because it is the farthest point from the axis of rotation: the momentum of lateral rotary force is the greatest and the medial back corner MBC is 'ready for action' (p. 20) as soon as a demand is made. The posterior horn of the medial meniscus PHMM serves as a 'latch' (p. 45).

---

53 Anterior drawer AD lateral rotation LR = ADLR.

54 The movement of the medial femoral condyle to the rear and the medial tibial condyle to the front place the insertions of TCL further apart and increases its initial slant downward and forward: TCL can then stretch to its maximum by 'lying down'.

55 The design of some complete sliding prostheses is based on the principle of rotary stability.

56 The medial tibial tubercule is more anterior and higher than the lateral tibial tubercule.

57 The posterior drawer PD lateral rotation LR Test = PDLR and the reverse R pivot shift PS Test = RPS.

(2) The 'emergency brake' is slow and sure:

● The anterior cruciate ligament ACL provides initial assistance by using its stretching possibilities to allow necessary lateral rotation (p. 40): the anterior cruciate ligament ACL is freed through the rearward shift of the axis of rotation (p. 45) and can use its stretching possibilities in a wide lateral rotary sweep limited by the medial facet of the lateral femoral condyle LFC.

● The tibial collateral ligament is the second to provide assistance, and does so by being placed in the best position for stretching: the tibial collateral ligament TCL 'lies down'[54], wrapping around the medial tibial tuberosity.

● The intercondylar eminence offers double security: it is an intercalary formation that blocks the medial tibial condyle MTC[55], and its medial tibial tubercule MTT[56], blocks the medial femoral condyle MFC.

(3) The 'brake' that actually stops the movement is the posterior cruciate ligament PCL.

● The rearward movement of the tibia from the lateral tibial condyle LTC[57] is provided with less 'geared down braking' (Figure 3.33).

F. 3.34

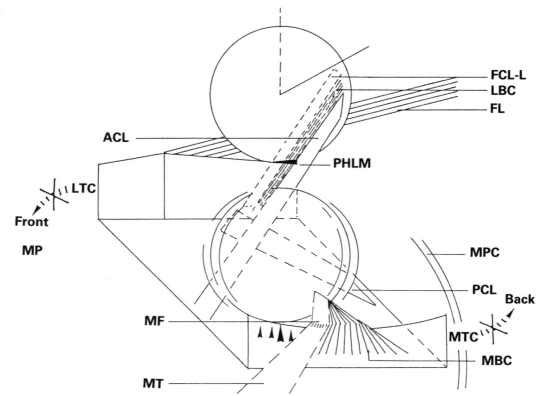

FCL-L
LBC
FL

ACL

PHLM

LTC

Front

MP

MPC

PCL

Back

MF

MTC

MBC

MT

F. 3.35

90°

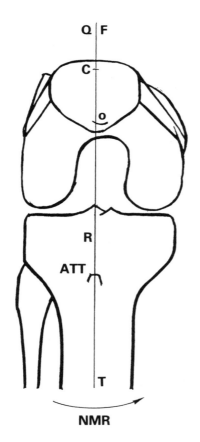

Q F

C

o

R

ATT

T

NMR

$Q\widehat{C}R = 180°$
$F\widehat{O}T = 180°$

F. 3.36

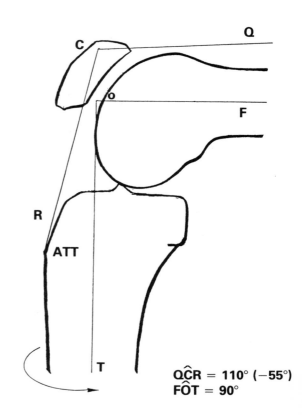

C

Q

o

F

R

ATT

T

$Q\widehat{C}R = 110° (-55°)$
$F\widehat{O}T = 90°$

(4) The 'main brake' is provided by the combination of the lateral back corner LBC and the anterior horn of the lateral meniscus.

- The lateral back corner LBC responds immediately for the same reasons as the MBC; its 'reinforcement' (p. 18 and Note 17) enabling it to support immediate demands.

- The anterior horn of the lateral meniscus AHLM serves as a 'latch' (p. 45).

The 'emergency brake' is provided by the fibular collateral ligament whose long head[58] places it in the best position for stretching: the fibular collateral ligament (long) 'lies down' in its normal orientation[59].

The 'brake' that actually stops the movement is the posterior cruciate ligament PCL which reinforces the activity of the lateral posterior capsule LPC.

In medial rotation MR, there is summary control (Figure 3.34). The forward movement of the tibia from the lateral tibial condyle LTC[60] is subjected to 'geared down braking':

(1) the 'main brake' is provided by the 'fragile' anterior cruciate ligament ACL (p. 17).

(2) the 'emergency brake' is gradual with three stages: The combined action of the lateral back corner LBC and the posterior horn of the lateral meniscus PHLM provides the initial assistance.

- The lateral back corner LBC responds immediately, and the control of forward movement of the lateral tibial condyle is never as rapid as control of rearward movement.

- The posterior horn of the lateral meniscus PHLM serves as a 'latch' (p. 46).

The fascia lata FL is the second component to provide assistance through its 'solid' terminal tendon (p. 27): the iliotibial aponeurosis, which can be partially assimilated with the fibular collateral ligament, is 'lying down' while the line of muscular force passes behind the centre of extension–flexion O with no more than 30° of flexion (p. 59).

The fibular collateral ligament is the third component to provide assistance, and does so through its long head FCL-L, repositioning itself in stretching position: the fibular collateral ligament (long) is once again 'lying down' but in the opposite direction[61].

(3) The 'brake' that actually stops the movement is the posterior cruciate ligament PCL.

The rearward movement of the tibia occurring at the medial tibial condyle MTC[62] has a rudimentary 'braking system' (Figure 3.34):

(1) The 'main brake' is provided by the medial back corner MBC but is not equipped with a latch, since the anterior horn of the medial meniscus does not participate (p. 46 Note 49).

(2) The 'emergency brake' is provided by the combined action of the meniscofemoral MF and the meniscotibial MT fibres (p. 15) but to a very limited extent.

(3) The 'brake' that actually stops the motion is the posterior cruciate ligament PCL, which reinforces the action of the medial posterior capsule MPC.

In 90° flexion in relation to 60° flexion (p. 49) (Figures 3.35 and 3.36): this is a sector of flexion that is not very useful, in addition to being dangerous because of the progressive destabilization that occurs: there is increased disalignment in a lateral view, more restricted free rotation, sliding double friction[63], and the loss of the central regulatory mechanism favours decoadaptation[64].

At the limit, complete flexion brings together the most unfavourable conditions in relation to complete extension (p. 35): the propensity for dislocation and the decrease to half of the support zone in terms of the smaller radii of the condylar spirals produces excessive constraints and leaves this position particularly vulnerable.

---

58 The short head integrates into the lateral back corner LBC (p. 19) and participates in the main braking effort, occasionally assisted by the popliteal muscle P (p. 30 and Notes 87, 90 and 93).

59 The movement of the lateral femoral condyle LFC to the front and the lateral tibial condyle LTC to the rear enables the insertions of the FCL-L (p. 18) to move further apart and to return to their initial slant downward and backward: the FCL-L can subsequently respond by stretching and 'lying down'.

60 The anterior drawer AD medial rotation MR Test = ADMR, and pivot shift PS Test = PS.

61 The movement of the lateral femoral condyle LFC toward the rear and the lateral tibial condyle LTC toward the front leaving the fibular collateral ligament (long) vertical at 30° of flexion (p. 44 and Note 42) and horizontal at 60°, with the insertions moving further apart and giving a new orientation, of slanting downward and forward: the fibular collateral ligament (long) by 'lying down' but in the opposite direction of the initial slant downward and to the rear.

62 The posterior drawer PD medial rotation MR Test = PDMR.

63 Pure sliding of both the femoral condyles (p. 38 and Note 25) and the tibial condyles (pp. 42 and 45; Notes 37 and 45) produces the conditions for skidding that is characteristic of the patellofemoral joint (p. 35 and Note 19).

64 The necessary medial rotation that enables the ACL and PCL to cross, creating coadaptation (p. 40) can no longer work: in fact the rearward movement of the femur is such that it is increasingly difficult to obtain interligamentous contact, and is impossible beyond 90° of flexion.

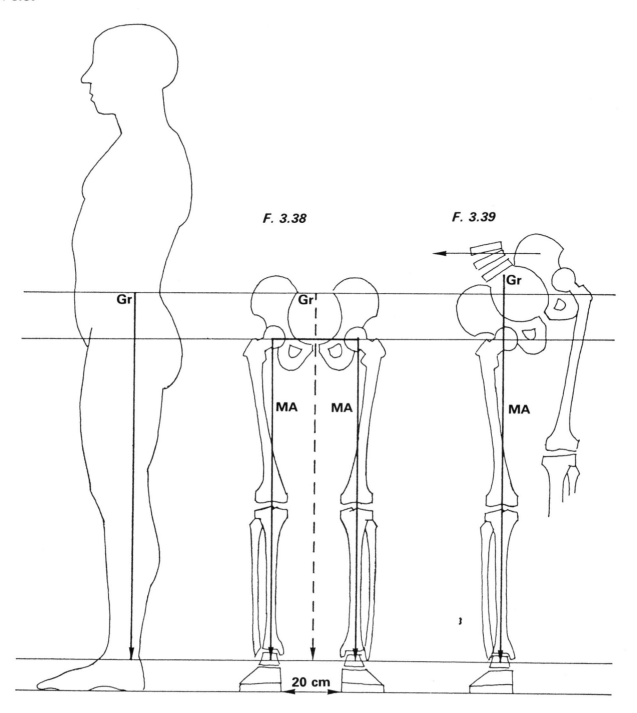

F. 3.37

F. 3.38

F. 3.39

Gr

Gr

Gr

MA   **MA**

MA

20 cm

Conclusion

The 'passive' knee is based on overall functional synergy, with continuous compromise between passive mobility and passive stability. The patellofemoral joint has a single degree of freedom, and is involved in a simple set of passive interactions. The tibiofemoral joint has two degrees of freedom, and is involved in a complex set of passive interactions; however, this joint is included in a functional unit and is capable of occasionally balancing out the forces involved in weight-bearing.

(1) The passive knee is an illustration of a single, inseparable functional unit. Unity requires a main function for each stabilizer and one or more secondary or emergency functions: this means that at 60° of flexion the ACL primarily keeps forward movement of the tibial intercondylar space in check (p. 46) as well as serving as the initial 'emergency brake' for forward movement of the medial tibial condyle (p. 47); the posterior cruciate ligament PCL primarily keeps in check the rearward movement of the tibial intercondylar space (p. 46), as well as being the 'real brake' for forward and rearward movement of the medial tibial condyle and lateral tibial condyle (pp. 47 and 49), and reinforcing lateral stability in extension (p. 38); the peripheral stabilizers must also be able to serve several functions, particularly the medial back corner MBC, which is the primary component keeping in check the forward movement of the tibial intercondylar space (p. 46) and the 'main brake' for the forward movement of the medial tibial condyle MTC (p. 47).

Lack of separation between the 'mobile' lateral compartment and the 'stable' medial compartment (p. 38) results from efforts at metering out and harmonizing actions that take place in the intercalary compartment (p. 38): the central structure acts as a pivot, favouring either mobility or stability, which is why it has received more picturesque names relating to its servomechanical functions, for example 'central pivot' and 'centre of the knee'.

(2) The balancing of weight-bearing (p. 32 and Note 2) can sometimes be carried out by a single 'passive' knee, the standing position offering a number of balanced variations, including some that are fundamental:

The motionless standing position is involved in balance when standing on one or both feet, but under the following conditions:

(a) Passive balance and extension occurs because:

● Extension makes it possible to lock the knee (p. 33).

● Passive balance in the absence of any muscular contraction makes it possible to direct the line of gravity Gr[65] through the mechanical axis of the tibiofemoral joint MA[66], to the extent that MA can be made vertical[67]: Gr can therefore be substituted for MA in the absence of any lateral constraint.

(b) Balance with support by two feet produces the 'at-ease' position[68], the mechanical axis of the tibiofemoral joint MA becoming vertical when the feet are spread approximately 20 cm apart (Figures 3.37 and 3.38): the line of gravity Gr passes through the mechanical axis of the tibiofemoral joint MA of the supporting lower limbs, dividing weight into two parallel and equal resultants.

(c) Balance with support by one foot attempts to maintain the acrobatic standing position, mechanical axis of the tibiofemoral joint MA is made vertical by swinging the trunk so that the lumbosacral joint is above the supporting hip (Figure 3.39): the line of gravity Gr passes through the mechanical axis of the tibiofemoral joint MA of the supporting lower limb, integrating the centre of gravity.

The upright position in movement involves support only on a single foot, and under the following conditions (Figure 3.40):

(a) The conditions relative to extension and biomechanical balance: Relative extension is attained in the sector of near extension, in other words in the direction flexion ZZ extension while the femur rolls forward (p. 40 and Note 26). Biomechanical balance uses energy provided by walking[69], making it fairly easy to direct the line of gravity Gr which it is slightly offset to the interior of the knee.

(b) The balance on one foot required by walking corresponds to the second stage or 'disengagement': a passive idle period that occurs between two active-passive working periods, corresponding at the very limit, to the transition from one of those periods to the other.

65 The line of gravity Gr is always represented by a vertical line corresponding to the projection of the centre of gravity into the area of foot support.

66 The mechanical axis of the tibiofemoral joint MA aligns three articular centres from the front and in profile: the centre of the head of the femur for the hip, the lateral tibial tubercule from the front and the pretibial space in the lateral view of the knee, the middle of the talus pulley for the ankle.

67 Making the mechanical axis of the tibiofemoral joint MA vertical is included within the extension upward of the anatomical axis of the tibia T (p. 33 and Note 12).

68 The standing-at-ease position justifies its name by the minimum of fatigue that occurs in the absence of muscle contraction.

69 Movement from the rear position forward is programmed in three stages. ● Stage one, deceleration: the line of gravity Gr falls behind the heel, the approach of the heel makes it possible to reduce the energy required in the preceding step. ● Stage two, disengagement: the line falls directly on the ankle, with the transition assured by having the foot flat on the ground. ● Stage three, acceleration: the line of gravity Gr falls in front of the ankle, the lifting of the ankle making it possible to direct the following step while providing it with energy.

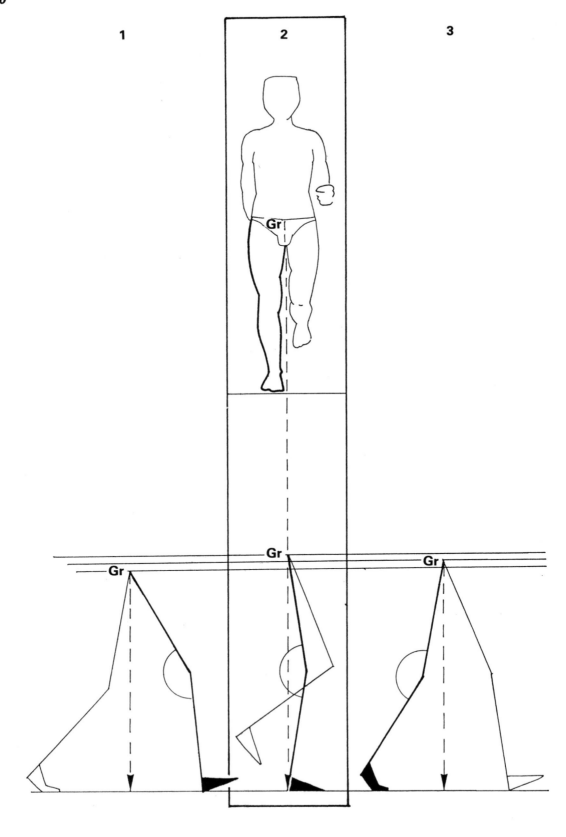

'Active knee'

Various sorts of voluntary participation of the muscle system occur, depending on whether that participation involves extension or flexion.

In *immobilization*, with two important features: only the tibiofemoral joint is involved, and the torque of active forces counterbalance one another to provide active stability[70].

In flexion, which makes movement possible, with two important features: both the patellofemoral joint with one degree of freedom and the tibiofemoral joint with two degrees of freedom are involved, and the interaction of forces results in torque that establishes a continuous compromise between active mobility and active stability[70].

An extremely demanding set of conditions is always required by muscle contraction and nearly always required by weight-bearing in the standing position; as a result the motor function operates with maximum constraints so that the knee's threshold of resistance can be reached or in certain cases exceeded[71].

'Active knee' in extension

The tibiofemoral joint is the only joint that participates in guaranteeing immobilization through active stability (p. 32), and this occurs through isometric muscle contraction[72].

The patellofemoral joint (Figures 3.41 and 3.42)

Although 'excluded' in extension, muscle activity at this joint nevertheless modifies the behaviour of the patella.

In relation to the 'passive' knee (p. 32):

- The action of the quadriceps enables the patella to exit from the trochlea and to occupy its highest position in the supratrochlear fossa[73].

- By spreading its force out horizontally, on the basis of front and lateral disalignment of the extensor apparatus, the action of the quadriceps subjects the patella to lateral movement and anteroposterior pressure on the femur.

F. 3.41

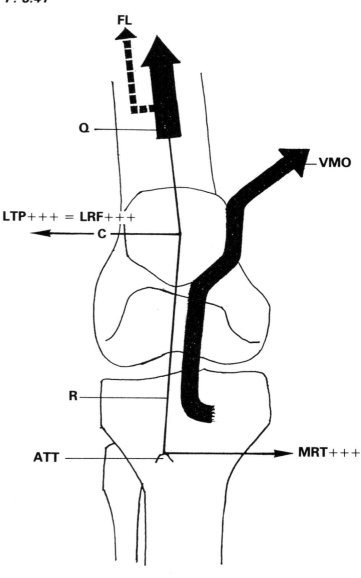

---

70 Ligamentoplasties occasionally rely on the principle of active stability which can help in the reduction or loss of passive stability caused by a sprain (p. 32 and Note 8) through tendinomuscular transfer: the transplant which is chosen and proportioned is active/passive, passive through the stretching of the tendon and active through the contraction reflex of the muscle body when stretched.

71 The knee's threshold of resistance will be reached or exceeded by a combination of factors, among which are the following: ● Minimum constraints of the passive knee limited to traction (inertia, outside manoeuvres). ● Submaximum constraints of the active knee, not only linked to traction (muscle contraction and weight-bearing) but also to pressure (counteracting weight-bearing and reaction to ground). ● Supermaximum constraints of occupation due, among other things, to carrying heavy loads. ● Critical constraints of certain sports (soccer, rugby, handball, basketball, track and field, and so forth), and the requirements of high performance (high level competition).

72 Isometric contraction contributes to immobilization, because the length of the muscle remains constant.

73 The apex of the patella is located 2–3 cm above the tibiofemoral interline.

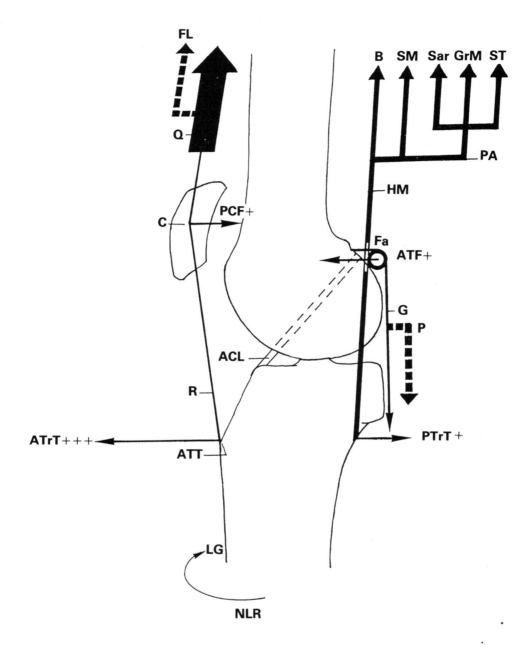

In the frontal plane (Figure 3.41) the force of lateral translation of the patella LTP +++ is highest in extension because it is inversely proportional to the angle QCR, which is narrowest from the front, and which is controlled by the vastus medialis (oblique) VMO.

In the sagittal plane (Figure 3.42), the patellar compression of the femur PCF + is lowest in extension because it is inversely proportional to the angle QCR, which is widest in a lateral view, resisting the weak forward thrust of the patella, which can no longer move laterally although it is no longer confined by the trochlea.

Tibiofemoral joint (Figures 3.41 and 3.42)

This is the only joint participating in extension, with muscle action reinforcing existing passive stability.

In relation to the 'passive' knee (p. 32): the quadriceps spreads its force out horizontally on the basis of frontal and lateral disalignment of the extensor apparatus, consequently developing lateral rotary force at the femur, medial rotary force and anterior traction at the tibia.

In the frontal plane (Figure 3.41) there are two opposing, parallel and superimposed forces that are greatest in extension, being inversely proportional to the angle QCR, which is narrowest in the frontal plane. The superior force is lateral rotary force of the femur LRF +++[74], which passes through the patella, but by lateral movement so that the forces LTP +++ and LRF +++ become similar. The inferior force arises from the anterior tibial tuberosity ATT, and is the medial rotary force of the tibia MRT +++[75]. Both combine for final control over lateral rotation of the tibia (p. 32). In the sagittal plane (Figure 3.42), the force of anterior traction of the tibia ATrT +++ is highest in extension, in relation to the extreme posterior location of the ATT where it originates. In addition, it acts contrary to the weak force of posterior traction of the tibia PTrT +[76] developed by the hamstring muscles HM, in other words by the biceps B, semimembranous muscle SM, pes anserinus PA which consist of the sartorius muscle Sar, gracilis muscle GrM and semitendinous muscle ST.

F. 3.43

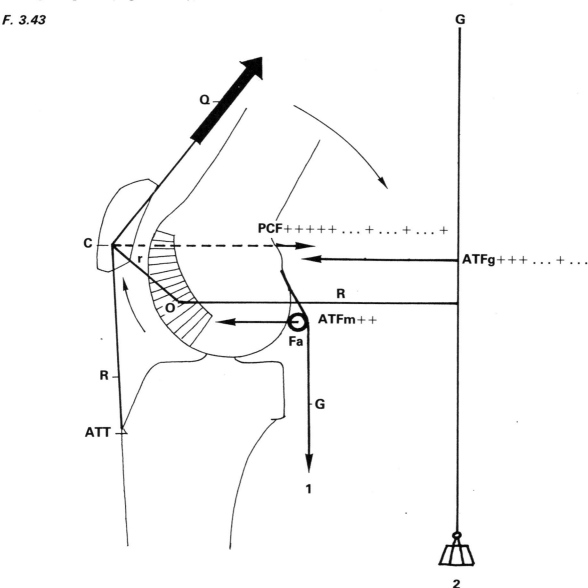

---

74 The force LRF +++ and its equivalent, the force LTP +++, arise essentially from the vastus lateralis VL.

75 The force MRT +++ basically depends on the muscle vastus medialis (oblique), which acts on the tibia by directly stretching the vastus medialis (p. 23) while also controlling the force LTP +++; the vastus medialis (oblique) can thereby be considered as neuroelectrically active as the other heads of the quadriceps.

76 The posterior constraints PC of the 'active' knee consist of the anterior thrust of the femur ATF and the posterior traction of the tibia PTT, whose low values in extension are going to increase in flexion.

On the whole, the 'active' knee relies on the guarantee of maximum stability, with active control providing a bolting down in the extended position.

In relation to the 'passive' knee (p. 32) active control essentially occurs at two points of application in the extensor apparatus.

The extensor apparatus (pp. 23–25) is the basic element in active control because of the quadriceps Q, assisted by the fascia lata FL. The torque of forces LRF-MRT checks lateral rotation of the tibia (p. 33). The vastus medialis (oblique) VMO controls the force of lateral translation of the patella LTP. The combination of forces PCF + ATrT controls the posterior constraints PC = ATF + PTrT.

The two essential points of application consist of the functional centre of the patella C and the anterior tibial tuberosity ATT; the first forms the focal point of three controlling forces LRF, VMO and PCF, confirming its role as a sesamoid bone (p. 12); the second concentrates the two controlling forces MRT and ATrT, playing its role as the apophysis of traction.

The lower limb attains its extended position by being both straight and stiff, in other words the leg is stretched to its maximum at the hip, but actively, the stretching of the gastrocnemius muscle providing posterior reinforcement for the posterior capsule (p. 34).

'Bolting down' is guaranteed by intra-articular rigidity and confined to 'locking'.

There is complete rigidity in the central structure because the posterior cruciate ligament PCL has already been stretched by the 'passive' knee, and the anterior cruciate ligament ACL is, in its turn, stretched to its maximum by the 'active' knee as a result of the force of anterior traction of the tibia ATrT developed by the quadriceps. This exerts its greatest force in extension; the torque of the quadriceps/anterior cruciate ligament Q-ACL is predominantly active because of the quadriceps.

'Mechanical locking' provides no outlet for excessive constraints, a situation that results in at least three possibilities: the knee 'resists' but at the cost of a fracture of the upper quarter of the tibia; the knee is struck at its 'weak point' leaving an isolated lesion of the anterior cruciate ligament ACL (p. 17); or the knee 'breaks' at the levels of one of its connections, producing a more or less extensive meniscal, capsular and ligamentous lesion.

'Active knee' in flexion

The patellofemoral and tibiofemoral joints contribute to movement through active torque (p. 32); dynamic contraction[77] develops muscular force that mobilizes[78] and stabilizes[79].

The patellofemoral joint

This joint has only one degree of freedom, with a simple 'active' interaction.

In relation to the 'passive' knee in flexion (p. 35) and according to the direction of movement:

In extension flexion ZZ while the trochlea slides from bottom to top the following considerations apply.

(a) Active mobility calls into play the gastrocnemius muscle and weight-bearing as the price paid for increasing posterior constraints. Mobilization of the gastrocnemius muscle G is immediate but imposes certain constraints (Figure 3.43). The immediate muscle response arising essentially in the lateral head of the gastrocnemius muscle makes it possible to initiate flexion through the intermediary of the fabella Fa[80] while the line of gravitational force Gr falls in front or passes through the centre of extension-flexion O. Mobilizing muscle force increases with flexion but requires an initial muscular component of the force of forward thrust of the femur ATF m + +.

Mobilization by gravity Gr is secondary but imposes even more constraints (Figure 3.43). Weight-bearing takes over as soon as the line of gravitational force Gr falls behind the centre of extension-flexion O. Mobilizing gravitational force increases with flexion[81], but at the cost of a second gravitational component of the force of forward thrust of the femure ATF g + + + . . . + . . . + . . . +.

---

77 Dynamic contraction produces movement through variations in the length of the muscle.

78 Mobilizing muscular force is developed through so-called concentric dynamic contraction: muscle length shortens and muscle insertions come closer together.

79 Stabilizing muscular force is developed through so-called eccentric dynamic contraction: muscle length increases and muscle insertions move further from one another.

80 The fabella Fa bears on the lateral femoral condyle LFC (p. 26 and Note 25) below the centre of the extension-flexion O.

81 Mobilizing gravitational force benefits from the increase in leverage: in fact, the more the knee is flexed, the greater the leverage of R, the end of which is operated by body weight.

(b) Active stability calls the quadriceps Q into play at the patella.

Control over the force of lateral translation of the patella LTP, which is exclusively exercised by the vastus medialis (oblique) VMO, is released at the initiation of flexion. As soon as the patella is engaged in the trochlear pulley, it can press against a restraint in the form of the lateral facet of the trochlea LFT (Figure 3.44).

F. 3.44

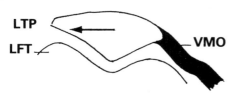

Control of flexion by the quadriceps increases as soon as flexion is initiated, in order to contain posterior constraints (Figure 3.43). Posterior constraints PC increase with flexion through the force of forward thrust of the femur, which is initially muscular and secondarily gravitational ATFm→ZZ g.

The stabilizing muscle force, developed by the quadriceps at the functional centre of the patella C, is represented by the impressive patellar compression on the femur PCF + + + + + + . . . + . . . + . . . + that depends on quadriceps Q force, which increases with flexion in order to provide the most economical use. The quadriceps Q force being proportional to the leverage R that represents the thickness of the patella-trochlear pulley, the increase up to 'full power' relies on the rolling of the trochlear spirals whose radii increase (p. 11) as flexion increases. Economic utilization of quadriceps Q force is rendered possible by rearward movement of the patella and femur (Figure 3.8), which attenuates the narrowing of the QCR angle[82] and,

by this fact, limits any rash increase in the patellar compression on the femur PCF[83].

In flexion ZZ extension while the trochlea is sliding from top to bottom:

Active mobility calls the quadriceps into play at the patella (Figure 3.41). The muscle response of the four heads (p. 23) is not equal: the vastus intermedius VI, the vastus lateralis VL and the vastus medialis (longitudinal) VML are equally active while the rectus femoris RF is less so[84]. The mobilizing muscle force increases with extension[85] while the resultant of Q force reconstitutes Q-ACL torque (p. 53).

Active stability calls the vastus medialis (oblique) and the gastrocnemius muscle into play (Figures 3.41 and 3.42). Control of force of lateral translation of the patella LTP, which is reserved for the vastus medialis (oblique) VMO, resumes at the approach of extension, since the patella can no longer press against the lateral facet of the trochlea. Control of extension by the gastrocnemius muscle G increases with the approach of extension[86].

Tibiofemoral joint

Having two degrees of freedom, the 'active' interaction is complex. In relation to the 'passive' knee in flexion (p. 37) interaction varies according to the direction of movement and the degree of freedom. In extension ZZ flexion (one degree of freedom), the tibia carries out necessary medial rotation NMR, controlled by the popliteal muscle P as soon as flexion is initiated[87].

(a) Active mobility relies on the double effect of the gastrocnemius muscle—weight-bearing (p. 56) and of a muscular reinforcement that requires new posterior constraints (Figure 3.45). The muscular reinforcement comes from the fascia lata FL[88] and particularly the hamstring muscles HM, in other words the biceps B, semimembranous musle SM

---

82 The decrease in the QCR angle is always less than would be anticipated for the angle of flexion: 25° for 30° of flexion (Figure 3.20), 45° for 60° (Figure 3.28), 55° for 90° (Figure 3.36), etc.

83 Increase in the patellar compression on the femur PCF is estimated at 40° of the Q force at 30° of flexion, decreasing to 75% instead of 80% at 60° of flexion, to 110% instead of 120% at 90° of flexion, etc. which is equivalent to saying that the QCR angle primarily reflects the reserve power of the quadriceps at 30° and 60° of flexion, subsequently eliminating the risk of crushing cartilaginous surfaces at 90° of flexion and beyond.

84 The rectus femoris RF, being the only part of the quadriceps that crosses two joints, cannot simultaneously flex the hip and extend the knee.

85 Insufficient extension of the leg is the inevitable consequence of any decrease in mobilizing quadriceps force: in fact, two-thirds of the force that it develops is used in the approach to extension.

86 The control of extension could possibly be reinforced by the rectus femoris RF, whose eccentric contraction might act like a strap. This would mean an alternation of rapid concentric (active mobility) with eccentric contraction (active stability) and could explain the frequency of lesions to the rectus femoris by 'mistaken automatism' in the approach to extension.

87 The popliteal muscle P is called into play in contraction at the initiation of flexion. It is the motor force of necessary medial rotation NMR: in fact, its nearly horizontal orientation and its simultaneously low and anterior position of its femoral attachment (pp. 30-31) provides a medial rotary effect making it easier for the knee to 'unscrew'.

88 The fascia lata FL works in a synergistic relationship with the biceps B by becoming a flexor-lateral rotator at around 30° of flexion, in other words as soon as the line of muscle force moves behind the centre of extension/flexion O.

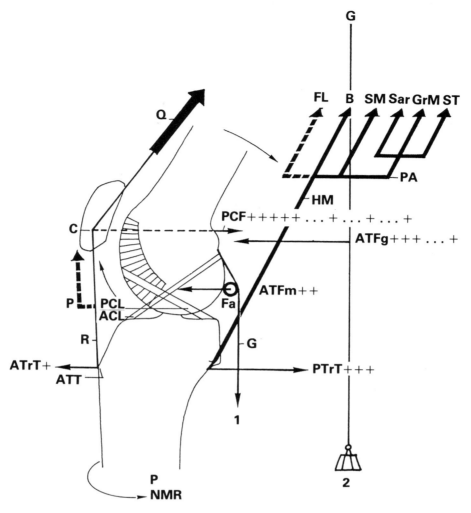

especially through its straight head and the pes anserinus muscles PA. Mobilizing muscular force increases with flexion but at the cost of increasing force of posterior traction of the tibia PTrT +++.

(b) Active stability relies on the action of the quadriceps that participates not only at the patella (p. 57), but also at the anterior tibial tuberosity and from reinforcement that is both muscular and ligamentous, in order to contain excess posterior constraints (Figure 3.45). Posterior constraints PC increase with flexion through the double muscular and gravitational force of forward thrust of the femur ATF mg and the force of posterior traction of the tibia. Stabilizing muscular force, developed in the quadriceps at the apophyseal point of application ATT, is represented by Q-ACL. It

depends on the force of anterior traction of the tibia ATrT, whose value decreases with flexion[89], contrary to the patellar compression of the femur (p. 57).

The stabilizing reinforcement is derived from both muscles and ligaments. Muscle reinforcement comes from the popliteal muscle P, which is called on as soon as flexion is initiated, with two synergistic effects occurring: the medial rotary effect providing indirect stabilization and enabling the cruciate ligaments to cross (p. 40), backed up by a directly stabilizing extensor effect[90].

Ligamentous reinforcement comes from the 'solid' posterior cruciate ligament PCL and acts primarily as the 'bolt' and the 'brake' (p. 51); the torque made

---

[89] Anterior traction of the tibia is greatest in extension ATrT +++ as a result of the more posterior location of the anterior tibial tuberosity ATT in relation to the patella (p. 56). It decreases in flexion, but in proportion to the rearward movement of the patella-femur, finally balancing out at 60° when the ATT is directly vertical to the patella (p. 36).

[90] The popliteal muscle P, which is called into play by contracting as soon as flexion is initiated, is not only a medial rotator but also an extensor: in fact, the anterior location of the femoral attachment (p. 30) could only emphasize flexion with rolling of the lateral femoral condyle (p. 38).

up of posterior constraints and the posterior cruciate ligament PC-PCL includes a dominant passive factor connected primarily with weight-bearing. In flexion ZZ extension (one degree of freedom), the tibia carries out necessary lateral rotation NLR under the influence of the lateral head of the gastrocnemius muscle LG as soon as extension is approached[91].

(a) Active mobility relies on the quadriceps (p. 53) as well as the action of the fascia lata FL which reinforces the quadriceps at the approach to extension[92] (Figure 3.42).

(b) Active stability relies on the gastrocnemius muscle (p. 56) and a double muscular reinforcement (Figure 3.42). The initial muscular reinforcement comes from the hamstring muscles HM, whose stabilizing muscular force reinforces that of the gastrocnemius muscle G, but far from extension. The second muscular reinforcement comes from the popliteal muscle P, whose stabilizing muscular force[93] reinforces that of the gastrocnemius muscle G, but only at the approach to extension.

In free rotation (two degrees of freedom), the tibia is subjected to lateral and medial rotation, but combined respectively with abduction or valgus Vl and adduction or varus Vr, the two opposing 'morphotypes' can be conceived as starting with the same muscle groups in demands that are preferential and antagonistic (Figures 3.46 and 3.47). The two 'morphotypes' are diametrically opposed, the first being called valgus Vl flexion F lateral rotation LR, the second being called varus Vr flexion F medial rotation MR. The demands are preferential no matter what 'morphotype' is involved, the predominant action being more lateral in the beginning of flexion and more rotary at the end of flexion[94].

The demands are antagonistic, according to the 'morphotype' considered.

(a) active mobility AM in valgus/flexion/lateral rotation VlFLR and active stability AS in varus/flexion/medial rotation VrFMR call upon a single

F. 3.46

$AM = FL + B$

Abd

$AS = Q + SM + PA$

VLF LR

F. 3.47

$AS = FL + B$

Add

$AM = Q + SM + PA$

VrF MR

posterolateral muscle group (p. 27) combining the fascia lata FL and the biceps B[95]. Up to 30°, the fascia lata FL is an extensor and produces valgus (p. 59 and Note 92). Beyond 30°, the biceps B, particularly the long part, imposes increasing lateral rotary movement with the aid of the fascia lata FL

---

91 The lateral head of the gastrocnemius muscle LG is the motor force of necessary lateral rotation NLR at the approach to extension: in fact, anterior thrust of the femur ATrF through the fabella Fa produces medial rotary momentum which, in its turn, is converted into lateral rotation of the tibia.

92 The fascia lata FL resumes its role as an extensor and a factor in valgus before 30° of flexion, in other words as soon as the line of muscle force moves in front of the centre of extension/flexion O.

93 The popliteal muscle P is called into play when stretched at the approach to extension, and may restrict the lateral compartment by tying it off: being in nearly horizontal position (p. 30), it is effectively in a good position to entwine and consequently make it easier to 'bolt down' the knee.

94 The verticalization and horizontalization of muscles that pass over two joints makes it possible to subject and support the knee to one predominant action: ● Verticalization in the beginning of flexion places those muscles in the role of guys that participate mostly in transverse action, in other words essentially lateral, and ● horizontalization at the end of the flexion places them in the role of providing traction and particularly producing rearward action, in other words essentially rotary and also increasing with flexion: in fact, the rearward movement of the axis of rotation (p. 42 and Notes 33 and 34) makes it possible to increase the momentum of the action and the rotary muscular force that results.

95 The participation of two muscles only provides rudimentary 'braking' of varus and medial rotation.

becoming a flexion and a lateral rotator (p. 57 and Note 88).

(b) active stability AS in valgus/flexion/lateral rotation VlFLR and active mobility AM in varus/ flexion/medial rotation VrFMR call upon two muscle groups, the anterosuperior group (pp. 23 and 24) and the posteromedial group (pp. 28–30) assembling the quadriceps Q, the three muscles of the pes anserinus PA and the semimembranous muscle SM[96]. Up to 30°, the quadriceps Q participates particularly in terms of two rotary forces, including lateral rotation of the femur and medial rotation of the tibia, both being increased in extension (p. 55) before decreasing and being counterbalanced in flexion, with alignment of the extensor apparatus. Beyond 30°, the semi- membranous muscle SM, particularly the reflected head and the pes anserinus muscles PA, take over from the quadriceps Q and impose increasing medial rotary movement.

Conclusion

The 'active' knee in relation to the 'passive' knee (p. 32) is also based on an overall functional synergy, a continuous compromise occurring between active mobility and active stabilization. The patellofemoral joint with one degree of freedom participates in a simple 'active' interaction. The tibiofemoral joint, with two degrees of freedom, participates in a complex 'active' interaction, but one that includes the whole functional unit and which is capable of counterbalancing weight-bearing at all times.

The functional unit is both unified and inseparable, as illustrated by the complementary relationship between muscles and ligaments, and can be demonstrated by two examples. The popliteal muscle appears in the role of a counterbalance for the intercalary compartment, with an 'active/ passive' compensatory mechanism, which is essential as soon as the knee arrives in the relatively unstable sector of initial mobility; this means that the 'unscrewing' effect of the popliteal muscle to initiate flexion (p. 58 and Note 90) is counter- balanced by the coadapting effect produced by the crossing of the ACL and the PCL (p. 40); on the other hand, the decoadapting effect produced by the uncrossing of ACL and PCL (p. 40) is compensated by the 'screw down' effect of the popliteal muscle at the approach to extension (p. 59 and Note 93). The proprioceptive reflex system is on continual alert:

96 Participation of five muscles provides for highly perfected 'braking' of valgus and lateral rotation.

F. 3.48

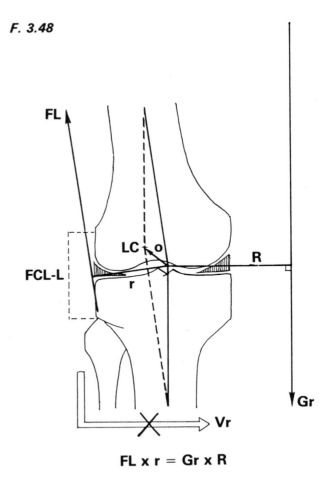

$$FL \times r = Gr \times R$$

the passive tendon, capsular and ligamentous apparatus is constantly sensing articular demands, the active muscular apparatus responds when demanded by so-called protective muscular contraction[97].

Weight-bearing can always be balanced by the 'active' knee[98], the standing position providing a large number of balanced variations including some that serve as references.

The immobile standing position involves single or two-footed support for balance, but under certain conditions, which involve extension and active/ passive equilibrium. *Extension* makes it possible to bolt down the knee (p. 56). *Active-passive equilibrium* with the aid of isometric muscle contraction (p. 53 and Note 72) makes it possible to direct the line of the force of gravity Gr through the

97 This tendinous, capsular and ligamentous vigilance is provided by receptors, in other words the endings and other spindles that maintain a permanent spy network on local-regional modifications: the 'sensations' received are methodologically arranged in an automatic motor response.
98 The muscle system can always control any tendency for the centre of gravity to slip outside of the area of foot support, but with a maximum of fatigue due to muscle contraction.

fascia lata FL backing up the fibular collateral ligament (long) FCL-L (Figure 3.48); the line of the force of gravity Gr can subsequently shift toward the interior of the knee, creating varus Vr stress. This is counterbalanced by the fibular collateral ligament (long) FCL-L that is called upon to stretch, and particularly by the fascia lata FL which is called upon to stretch at the cost of minimum lateral constraints LC[99].

Balance on two feet produces a standing 'at attention' position, in which it is always necessary to lock the ankles[100] in order to make it easier to place the trunk in a slightly inclined forward position (Figures 3.49 and 3.50): the line of force of gravity Gr is slightly in front of rather than being exactly vertical to the ankles. In other words, it is exactly in the middle of the foot support area, security in equilibrium being brought about by the division of weight and its distribution over a larger area.

In equilibrium on a single foot in the standing position[101], the shift of the lumbosacral joint of the supporting side must always be coordinated with slight adduction Add of the lower limb (Figure 3.51): the line of force of gravity Gr falls on the medial part of the instep of the foot, with balance becoming precarious because weight is not divided and is distributed over a reduced area.

F. 3.49

F. 3.50

F. 3.51

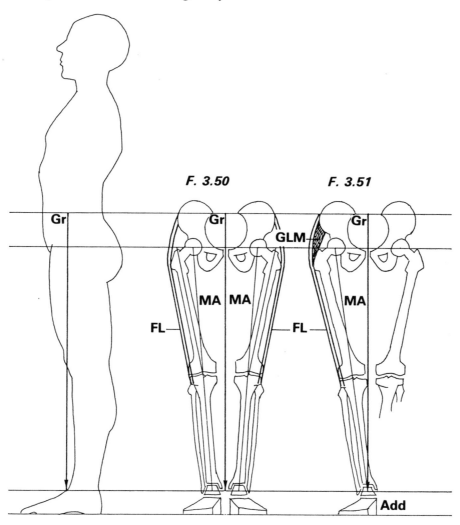

99 The parallelogram of forces including the Gr and FL demonstrates the lateral constraints LC with a resultant orientated outward and slightly upward (Figure 3.48).
100 The feet being solidly fixed to the soil and the legs firmly held in place by the posterior guys, the ankles can be locked in order to avoid flexion caused by weight-bearing.

101 The pelvis, which is controlled by the gluteus muscles GlM on the supporting side, is made horizontal or inclined: horizontal in the position where the non-supporting leg is flexed at the knee and only supports its own weight; inclined in the standing-at-ease position with lowering of the relieved side, the lower limb thereby freed to rest in slight passive flexion while being suspended from the hip and in contact with the ground.

The standing position in movement[102] only involves single foot support and under certain conditions (Figures 3.52 and 3.53), flexion and biomechanical equilibrium are called into play. Flexion creates the movement, and provides better balance by lowering the centre of gravity[103]: biomechanical equilibrium uses energy provided by movement, making it possible to direct a major part of the line of force of gravity Gr, while this force is increasingly shifted toward the interior of the knee with flexion[104].

The balance on a single foot required during walking (p. 51 and Note 69) initially corresponds to deceleration and subsequently to acceleration, in other words two full-time active-passive stages providing a multitude of balanced positions in reference to the two morphotypes chosen (p. 59); valgus flexion/lateral rotation VlFLR and varus flexion/medial rotation VrFMR provide more choice, since they are based, among other factors, on speed, change of direction toward or away from the support foot.

F. 3.52

F. 3.53

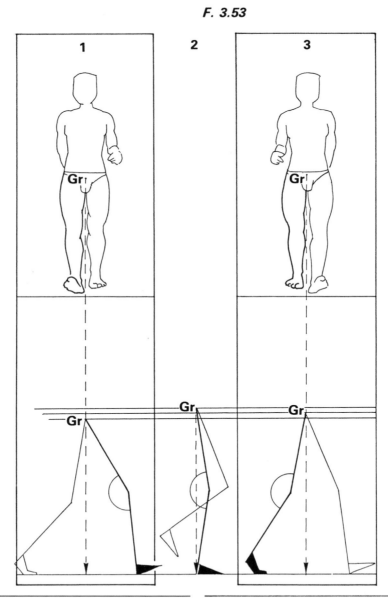

---

102 Walking takes place in two steps, the free step and the support step: ● the free step enables the corresponding lower limb to complete its oscillatory pace. ● the support step enables the corresponding lower limb to carry out its support phase where there is an alternation between double support and single foot support, the latter posing a real problem of balance.

103 Security of balance is as much a function of increasing the support area as of lowering the centre of gravity.

104 The dependence on biomechanical energy explains why it is less tiring to walk quickly than slowly.

Chapter 4

DIAGNOSTIC SIGNS & SYMPTOMS

The knee constitutes a single, inseparable functional unit, and only systematic coordination of the various types of investigation can provide a basis for diagnosis and assessment of lesions.

For examination of the knee—a check-list can be drawn up, which nearly always provides a definite pointer to the correct diagnosis.

Interview

A lengthy interview is carried out in order to provide complete and detailed information concerning the features listed below.

Patient identification

- Age, sex and weight/height ratio.
- Occupation.
- Athletic activity—sports engaged in; position occupied in team games; occasional, regular or high level participation.
- Any personal or family history related to the locomotor system[1].

Reasons for the consultation

There are four possible categories of complaint, although combinations occur:

- Knee pain.
- Stiffness or slipping of the knee.
- Abnormal size (increased or reduced) or positioning of the knee.
- Weakness of the knee, reflected in instability, episodes of dislocation or failure which may result in falls.

Key events

- Spontaneous onset will have usually occurred some time ago and will not usually have been severe.
- A provoked onset is more often recent and dramatic: a mechanism is triggered with or without outside contact[2] and details must be gathered concerning four essential aspects: whether the knee was bent or straight; whether or not it was supporting the patient's weight; whether the impact was direct or distant, and the site of the impact[3]. The severity[4] must be assessed on the basis of three signs occurring at the time of the initial accident: 'syncopal' pain, snapping sound[5] and immediate, total incapacity resulting, for athletes, in the player's leaving the field.
- Diagnostic and therapeutic measures adopted at the the time.
- Subsequent history, in terms of three categories—acute with crises, subacute with recurrent episodes, chronic and stable.

Extent of disability[6]

This must be assessed in three areas: ordinary activity in everyday life; the normal requirements of work; and athletic activity under conditions of training or competition.

The mechanism of injury[7] involves loading, or overloading, usually involving a single position, movement or gesture. The activity involves one of the following:

- Kneeling, squatting, prolonged sitting in a vehicle or cinema, arising, weight-bearing on the affected knee only.
- Going up or down stairs or a slope.

---

1 The clearest memories are those such as 'synovial effusion', a plaster cast, abnormal gait during childhood, episodes of locking, dislocation, sprain or a 'blow received'.

2 The trigger mechanism supposes excessive kinetic force, of either endogenous (some mechanism not involving contact) or exogenous (a mechanism involving contact) origin, with which the knee is unable to cope.

3 The visible point of impact in the form of a bruise or wound of the soft tissues is usually on the anterior or lateral surface of the knee or on the inner surface of the foot.

4 Severity signifies a loss of continuity within the menisco-capsulo-ligamentous system, due to tearing or disinsertion, and within the tendino-muscular system, due to rupture.

5 The 'snap' is felt, and sometimes heard, like the snapping of a taut string. This means that the ripping or disinsertion of the menisco-capsulo-ligamentous system is equivalent to the fracture of a bone or rupture of the tendino-muscular system.

6 Assessment of the loss of functional capacity is based primarily on the subject's description.

7 The mechanism of injury includes indicative mechanical factors described as predisposing, triggering or aggravating.

- A specific amount of walking (given distance or duration), with or without claudication, with or without crutches, on level and then uneven ground, when hurrying, when carrying heavy objects, etc.—Running over medium or long distances, or sprinting, changes of direction cutting towards or away from the affected side, taking-off or landing when jumping, etc.

The most frequent causes include the following.

Pain, which can be defined on the basis of three parameters:

- The site of involvement, whether anterior, lateral or posterior, and vertical, horizontal or at a specific point.
- Intensity—acute, moderate or merely a nuisance.
- The daily pattern of mechanical[8], inflammatory[9] causes, or their combination.

The defects, are divided into two categories.

Stiffness[10], which may or may not reduce the functional range of movement[11] or may be superceded by ankylosis[12], and two types of sliding defect[13]: abnormal sound—a dry, cracking sound is less significant than an acute, painful creaking—and locking or pseudolocking[14], which are characterized by sudden appearance and reduction and by the possible association with immediate, audible return[15].

Deformity, which may take three forms:

- An abnormal position, usually flexed.
- A general or local swelling, which may be recurrent or permanent or
- A persistent reduction in the segmental volume.

Failing of the knee may be manifested under three identical types of circumstances, that the patient may be able to demonstrate:

- Instability[16] which may be described in various ways: 'My knee floats, slips, isn't solid, can't be relied on, isn't dependable . . . gives, turns or twists . . . I've lost confidence in it', etc.
- Giving way[17].
- Dislocation[18] which is usually spectacular. In the patellofemoral joint, there is an audible click-clack sound due to external dislocation of the patella[19]. In the tibiofemoral joint, there is an associated pivot shift of the lateral tibial condyle (p. 74).

Clinical Examination

The clinical examination should be carried out under the most suitable conditions i.e. with the patient sufficiently undressed[20] to allow comparison of the affected side with the normal one, and observation not only of the knee joint, but of the joints above and below it.

Observation

The observation is carried out with the patient standing (Figures 4.1–4.6).

The examination with the weight on both feet is carried out against a vertical surface with legs touching[21] and feet parallel, first in the 'at ease' position, and then 'at attention' (pp. 51 and 61).

---

8 The pain occurs during the daytime, becoming more severe towards evening, due to sustained exertion and tiredness, and reduced by rest and by putting the feet up.

9 Here the pain occurs at night, waking the patient up during the second half of the night, and sometimes at a regular time; the pain fades after limbering up in the morning.

10 The stiffness is the subjective perception of active or passive limitation of the amplitude of the joint.

11 The functional arc extends from complete extension to 100° of flexion, and permits virtually normal everyday activity and even some occupational activities.

12 The ankylosis is complete i.e. osseous and irreversible; this leaves the knee stiff.

13 Sliding defects combine a whole series of disturbances caused by abnormal contact of the articular surfaces. The intra-articular causes are many, and include an obstacle, an alteration in the cartilaginous area, or a foreign body.

14 'True' locking is different from transient, 'pseudo'-locking.

15 The immediate audible rebound accompanies the return to normal contact between the joint surfaces.

16 Instability is the subjective awareness of the excessive mobility produced by a menisco-capsulo-ligamentous lesion.

17 Giving-way results from loss of reflex active/passive control without any loss of normal articular alignment.

18 Dislocation results from loss of active/passive control and includes articular disorder, either subluxation or full dislocation.

19 The first and second 'click-clack' sounds result from the lateral dislocation of the patella and its subsequent reduction; this sequence results in a double blow against the external surface of the tibiofemoral joint (p. 36).

20 The patient should be examined wearing underpants without shoes or socks.

21 The legs touch at the ankles in the case of genu varus, and at the knees in the case of genu valgum.

The following are observed in frontal view:

- Any inequality of the length of the legs due to tilting of the pelvis or curvature of the spine e.g. with the downwards tilt and convexity above the shorter leg[22].
- Genu varum GVr[23] or genu valgum GVl[24].

The following are particularly observed in lateral view:

- Any increase in the lumbar curvature, which could be related to excessive anteversion of the neck of the femur.
- Genu flexum GFx or genu recurvatus GRv.

The podoscope is used to investigate for signs of hollow foot, or the valgus flat foot known as physiological valgus flat foot, i.e. the foot when a child begins to walk. This may be a cause of anxiety to parents if it persists, and special soles may be used to treat it.

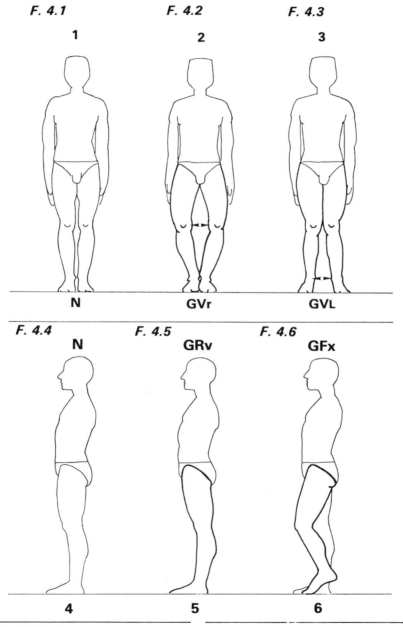

F. 4.1   F. 4.2   F. 4.3

1   2   3

N   GVr   GVL

F. 4.4   N   F. 4.5   GRv   F. 4.6   GFx

4   5   6

22 Pelvispinal compensation is abolished when seated.
23 Genu varum is apparent from the gap between the knees when the insides of the ankles touch.

24 Genu valgum is apparent from the gap between the ankle bones when the insides of the knees touch.

Analysis of the gait essentially consists of determining the angle of stepping[25] and identification of any limp. Increased angle of stepping in an abnormal gait may be obvious, with the feet turned outwards in a 'duck walk' or may be dissimulated, for appearance's sake. Minor limping may be heard rather than seen, as a shuffling avoidance of a painful step; a major amount of limping may accompany ankylosis in extension[26] and even more in flexion[27].

The examination

This is carried out with the patient lying in the dorsal decubitus position on a hard surface with a head-rest; the arms are laid along the body, the legs stretched out alongside each other, but attempting to overcome pelvis-spinal compensation[28].

Visual inspection

The legs are compared in order to detect the presence of any of the following:

An unnatural position, usually flexed.

Swelling, which may be restricted to the bulge of prepatellar hygroma, retraction due to tendino-muscular rupture, trapped effusion from the suprapatellar fold, meniscal or popliteal cyst; or diffuse, with the formation of a crescent-shaped swelling (concave side downwards) above the patella and obliteration of the lateropatellar hollows indicating widespread effusion.

Loss of volume, essentially linked to muscle wasting and particularly obvious along the vastus medialis.

Immediate reddening[29]; delayed ecchymosis which is somewhat lopsided, due to gradual infiltration of haemarthrosis which empties spontaneously through a breach in the capsular and ligamentous structure, or of the haematoma resulting from tendinomuscular 'snapping', or one that indicates having been 'kneed' at the site of direct violence.

Scar of surgical or traumatic origin, ridges or 'peau d'orange' due to infiltration of cellulitis, varices, etc.

Palpation

The legs are compared in extension and then in flexion.

When extended in the dorsal decubitus position, any transverse mobility of the patella indicates muscular laxity. The following features are noted.

The exact site of pain: deep palpation of the patella can explore the medial and lateral facets[30] for any cartilaginous lesions (see Figure 4.8); superficial palpation can locate normal or ectopic points of pain. Normal painful points follow interlines[31], the sites of suprapatellar and infrapatellar attachments and the tibiofemoral tubercule attachments. Ectopic points of pain may occur on the operated knee; this usually involves scar neuroma of the patellar branch of the saphenus or inflammatory granuloma along nylon suture along the ridges of the femoral condyles.

- Heat, detected using the back of the hand.
- Cellulitic infiltration, detected by pinching and pressing.
- Muscle consistency, in terms of tonicity and trophicity.
- Induration of a lateral meniscal cyst, an arthrophyte, the taut string of the plica, the thickening of a prepatellar hygroma or synovial lipoma.
- Widespread effusion detected by frontal patellar impact (Figure 4.9)[32].

---

25 There is an angle between the direction of walking and the longitudinal axis of the footprint drawn between the heelprint and the space between the prints of the second and third toes. The angle opens forwards and outwards and is usually between 10° and 15°. (see Figure 4.7).

26 Ankylosis in extension, or in the functional position, is often well coped with; the stiffness which occurs during stretching can be compensated by equinus-type foot position, which causes little inconvenience since it occurs on the 'good' side.

27 Ankylosis in flexion, on the other hand, is difficult to cope with; the rigidity experienced in contraction must be compensated for by equinus-type foot position, but this is highly inconvenient since it occurs on the same side as the knee injury.

28 Correction is intended to reduce the lumbar curvature by forcing the spinous processes into contact with the hard surface and by bringing the anterosuperior iliac crests into line both vertically (or transverse to the plane of observation) and horizontally (or in parallel to the plane of viewing).

29 The redness caused by ice packs may be misleading!

30 The 'hidden face' of the patella can only be exposed by extension during partial eversion in the supratrochlear fossa (p. 33).

31 Examination for the 'squeal' of the meniscus, by pressure on the interline and by manoeuvres involving lateral pressure, may often provide decisive diagnostic evidence.

32 The patella is jammed against the tibiofemoral joint, resulting in characteristic impact; the patella is previously raised by shunting the contents of the synovial pouches beneath the patella (p. 14).

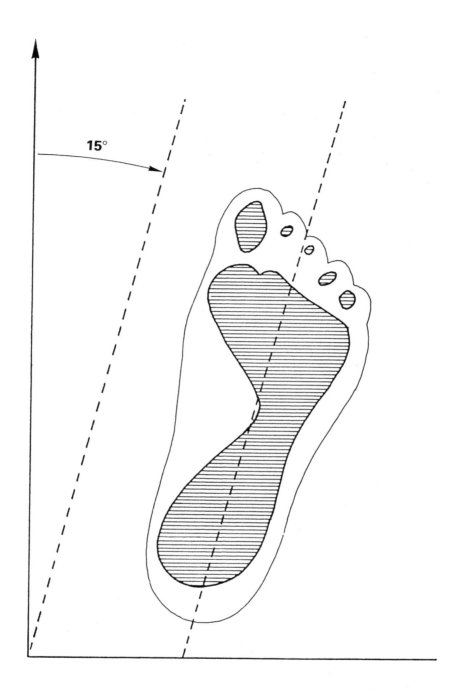

15°

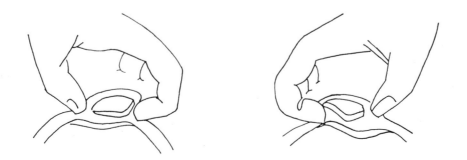

- Exaggeration of bayonet deformity[33] due to frontal patellar imbalance resulting from increased frontal disalignment of the extensor apparatus (see Figure 4.10).
- Absence of inguinal or retrocrural adenopathy.

When flexed in the ventral decubitus position the leg is held in order to obtain relaxation of the muscles, making it possible to investigate the following (Figure 4.11):

- painful points around the joint as flexion begins.
- deep pain of the femoral condyle-bearing surface at 60° of flexion.
- filling of posterior bursitis or popliteal cyst at 90° of flexion.

Active mobilization

This is performed with the patient in the dorsal decubitus position. Comparisons are made and joint range of movement, performance in active tests and muscular performance assessed.

Joint range of movement
The active range extends from 0° in extension[34] to 130° in flexion; during extension the patella is immobilized (p. 53), and during flexion between 30°and 60°, tibiofemoral rotation is 20° to 30°.

Active restriction due to the unnatural, but reducible, defence posture (p. 66) is a muscle reflex and produces slow and very painful stopping after running, followed by a sudden retreat to the original position. The reflex is triggered by pain and intensified by apprehension, usually resulting in a pain-avoiding flexion.

Active tests
Examination of the tibiofemoral joint is carried out to determine any imbalance of the patella. The patient's thigh is set against the bent knee of the examining physician, who thereby has both hands free and is able to use one to manipulate the patella.

The extension/flexion movement[35] reveals the following features:

- At the initiation of flexion, the overly high patella strikes the upper edge of the joint as it engages.
- At 30° of flexion and rotation O RO, nonalignment of the extensor apparatus (p. 41), such as persistence of the bayonet

F. 4.9

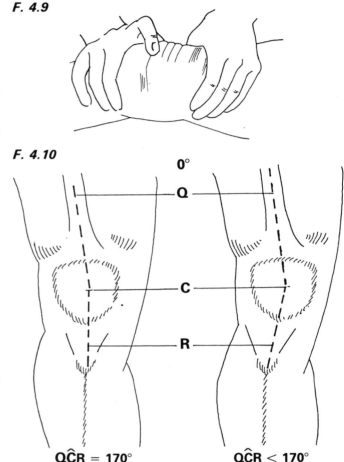

F. 4.10

QĈR = 170°   QĈR < 170°

F. 4.11

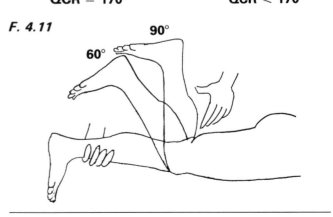

---

33 The bayonet formed by the quadriceps tendon QT, patella C and patellar tendon PT clearly leaves its mark by detaching itself from the ATT and the tibial crest; this deformity may be attenuated during extension due to lateral displacement of the patella in the supratrochlear fossa (p. 33 and Note 10).

34 This reference to 0° of extension is possible because a position is selected which is both anatomical and functional; the locking obtained offers a double guarantee of both straightness and stiffness and so confers maximum safety (p. 56).

35 The extension/flexion movement in dorsal decubitus is actively stabilized by means of the essential contribution of the quadriceps at its patellar and apophyseal points of application (pp. 56 and 58); this makes it possible to test the extensor apparatus under maximum effort.

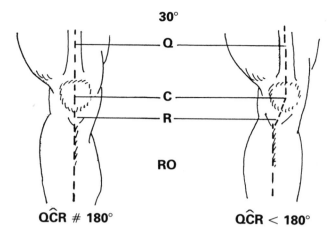

QĈR # 180°   QĈR < 180°

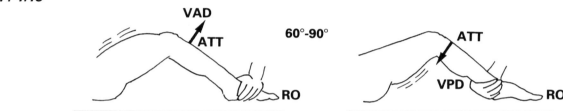

deformity (see Figure 4.12), confirms frontal imbalance[36].

● During the movement one hand is firmly pressed against the anterior surface of the patella; this may evoke abnormal sounds and, in particular, pain which is sufficiently severe to halt the movement in a position that indicates the site of the lesion[37].

Examination of the tibiofemoral joint is carried out to determine any abnormal movement signifying meniscal, capsular and ligamentous lesion. The leg is placed in 60° to 90° of flexion and rotation O RO and the examining physician observes the sequence of changes in the shape of the anterior tibial tuberosity ATT whilst holding the patient's foot flat with one hand.

Static or 'voluntary' tests involving isometric contractions deliberately produced by the patient include the following.

---

36 The bayonet deformity, which may be camouflaged by lateral subluxation of the patella and contraction of the quadriceps, becomes clearly apparent again at 30° of flexion as soon as the patella is manually recentered.

37 The point of contact of the patella varies on the basis of the angle of flexion (p. 36). At around 30° of flexion the lower third is in contact, at around 60° the middle third, at around 90° the upper third and above 90° the lateral margins of the articular facets and the third facet are brought into contact.

The voluntary anterior drawer sign VAD (see Figure 4.13): the patient exerts extension effort against resistance, essentially by bringing the quadriceps into play (p. 57). The VAD test is positive in the case of a lesion affecting both the anterior crucial ligament ACL and the medial back corner MBC (p. 47) or others. Abnormal mobilization in the anterior drawer sign, visible as the progressive emergence of the ATT, results from forward subluxation from the tibial intercondylar space while it disappears during relaxation.

The voluntary posterior drawer sign VPD (Figure 4.13). The patient flexes his knee against resistance, mainly by using the hamstring muscles (p. 59). The VPD test is positive in the case of a specific lesion of the posterior cruciate ligament PCL (p. 47); the abnormal mobility, seen in the posterior drawer sign as the ATT gradually disappears in posterior subluxation of the intercondylar space and may persist during relaxation.

Assessment of the musculature
Systematic muscle-by-muscle examination makes it possible to identify muscular lesion by reproducing the pain and evaluating the muscular deficiency.

Muscle wasting is determined from the maximum circumference of the thigh and calf at a given

F. 4.14

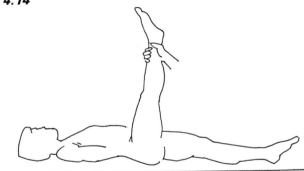

F. 4.15

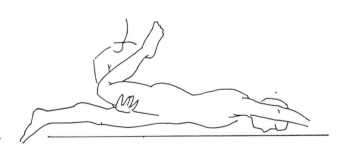

distance from the point or base of the patella, usually 15 cm in either direction.

Muscle strength is tested during isometric contraction[38], and scored successively:

● during extension; and

● during 30°, 60° and 90° of flexion with lateral or medial rotation, depending on whether it is the posterolateral (p. 27) or posteromedial group of the hamstring muscles.

Muscle elasticity is evaluated at peak stretch in suitable positions. In dorsal decubitus with the knee extended (see Figure 4.14), the hamstring muscles are selectively called into play at the limit of extension of the hip, i.e. at around 90°. In ventral decubitus, with the knee flexed (see Figure 4.15), the rectus femoris is selectively called into play at the limit of extension of the hip, i.e. at around 20°.

Passive mobilization

This is carried out with the patient in dorsal decubitus. The legs are compared after elimination of any defence reaction[39] and the performance in active tests and range of movement of the joint are assessed.

Joint range of movement
The passive range extends from beyond −10° during physiological recurvatum (p. 34) to 150° during heel-to-thigh[40]. When fully extended, the patella shows transverse mobility which is equal in medial and lateral directions (p. 34); when flexed at 30° or 60°, tibiofemoral rotation can attain 30° and 40° respectively.

Passive limitation due to an unnatural position with irreversible locking (p. 66) results in deficit.

Passive limitation after evacuation of effusion results in sudden, complete and immediate locking, accompanied by virtually no pain, at the end of the movement, with no return. This deficit may be either articular or periarticular, resulting in: reduced extension in meniscal lesion or posterolateral capsule and ligament retraction, producing irreversible flexum. Loss of flexion in cases of shortening of the extensor apparatus[41] or of anterolateral capsule and ligament retraction may pass unnoticed.

Increase in passive mobility may be either patellofemoral or tibiofemoral. During complete extension of the patellofemoral joint, transverse lateral hypermobility of the patella is a sign of a lesion of the medial patellar retinaculum.

In the case of the tibiofemoral joint, during complete extension, hyperextension HE occurs in cases of lesion to the posterior capsule LPC or MPC or to the posterior cruciate ligament PCL (p. 34); during 60° flexion, lateral hyperrotation LHR occurs in cases of associated lesion of the medial back corner MBC + anterior cruciate ligament ACL (p. 47) or of the lateral back corner LBC (p. 47) + popliteal muscle P (p. 59 and Note 93) or a combination of these lesions.

---

38 Isometric contraction is performed without any movement, the length of the muscle remaining unchanged.

39 Once osteoarticular fracture has been eliminated, aspiration of the haemarthrosis and general anaesthetic provide the best conditions under which to carry out examination of a 'fresh' sprain.

40 Reduction of the muscle mass in relaxation allows a greater degree of flexion.

41 This shortening of the extensor apparatus may have many causes, including fixing of the patella by the adherences of the quadriceps or of the subquadricipital bursa, lowering of the patella or of the anterior tibial tuberosity ATT or patella baja, etc.

Passive tests

Exploration of the extended patellofemoral joint consists of testing for the 'plane sign' (Figure 4.16)—longitudinal or transverse mobilization over the background detects lesion of the cartilage from a dry, painful rasping sound[42]. Examination of the femoral joint consists of looking for abnormal mobility indicative of meniscal, capsular and ligamentous lesion. The patient's thigh is set against a hard surface or against the bent knee of the examining physician, who is then able to carry out passive mobilization of the leg firmly but in a relaxed state and without causing pain.

Static tests of the extended knee.

- Valgus extension test VlE and varus extension test VrE. Forced, distal mobilization of the leg (see Figure 4.17) is obtained by grasping the lower quarter of the leg and producing or adduction.

The VlE test is positive in cases of an extensive lesion affecting at least the posterior cruciate ligament PCL, the tibial collateral ligament TCL and the medial back corner MBC (p. 35): abnormal mobility in valgus is due to internal lateral opening. The VrE test is positive in cases of an extensive lesion affecting at least the posterior cruciate ligament PCL, the long fibular collateral ligament FCL-L and the lateral back corner LBC (p. 35); the abnormal mobility of varus is due to external lateral opening.

- The drawer sign—extension test DE. Forced, proximal mobilisation of the leg (see Figure 4.18) is obtained by grasping the upper quarter and applying forwards/backwards pressure in rotation O as extension is approached.

The DE test is positive in lesions of the anterior cruciate ligament ACL or of the posterior cruciate ligament PCL: Abnormal mobility in the anterior or posterior drawer sign is due to anterior or posterior subluxation of the tibial intercondylar space[43].

- The big toe test BT. Forced, distal mobilization of the leg is obtained by picking up the leg by the big toe (see Figure 4.19); this has the advantage of producing a triple effect combining adduction, lateral rotation and recurvatum.

---

42 A painless 'plane sign' is frequent among healthy subjects and is of no diagnostic significance.

43 The extension drawer sign test DE is particularly useful in apprehensive patients. It is in fact an inexact test, which can detect abnormal mobility behind a defence reaction, but which lacks the mechanical precision of more specific tests.

F. 4.16

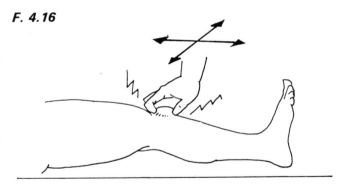

F. 4.17

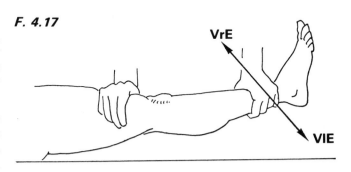

F. 4.18

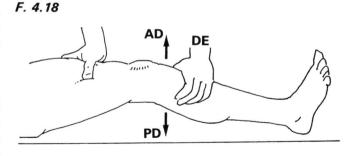

F. 4.19

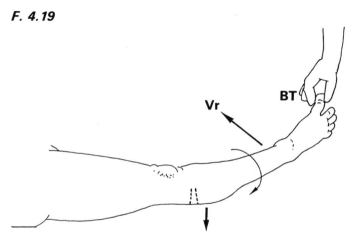

The BT is positive in an associated lesion of the lateral back LBC and the popliteal muscle P ± the posterior cruciate ligament PCL: the abnormal mobility of varus, with apparent fall of the tibia, corresponds to posterolateral opening and posterior subluxation of the lateral tibial condyle.

Static tests at 30° flexion.

Valgus lateral rotation VlLR and valgus medial rotation VlMR tests:

- Forced, distal mobilization of the leg (Figure 4.20) is obtained by grasping the heel and using abduction, then adduction during lateral rotation LR.

- VlLR or VlE is positive in lesion of the tibial collateral ligament TCL and of the medial back corner MBC (p. 44); the abnormal mobility of valgus is due to medial opening.

- The VrLR or VrE is positive in lesion of the long fibular collateral ligament FCL-L and of the lateral back corner LBC (p. 44); the abnormal mobility of varus is due to lateral opening.

Valgus medial rotation VlMR and varus medial rotation VrMR tests:

- Forced mobilization of the leg is carried out in a similar fashion (see Figure 4.20) but medial rotation is used MR.

- VlMR or VlE is positive in lesion of the medial back corner MBC affecting the posterior portion (p. 47); the abnormal mobility of valgus is due to medial opening.

- VrMR is positive in lesion of the lateral front corner LFc (p. 47); the abnormal mobility of varus is due to lateral opening.

Static tests at 60° and 90° flexion:

- Anterior drawer sign—rotation O ADRO, and anterior drawer sign—lateral rotation ADLR, and anterior drawer sign—medial rotation ADMR.

- Forced, proximal rotation of the leg (Figure 4.21) is obtained by grasping the upper quarter of the leg and using forwards pressure during rotation O RO, lateral rotation LR and then medial rotation MR. Rotation is applied from the foot, which is held flat by the examining physician.

- The ADRO test is positive in lesion of both the medial back corner LBC + the anterior cruciate ligament ACL (p. 46); abnormal

mobility of the anterior drawer sign is due to anterior subluxation of the tibial intercondylar space.

- The ADLR test is positive in extensive lesion affecting at least the medial back corner MBC, the posterior horn of the medial meniscus PHMM, the anterior cruciate ligament ACL and, in some cases, the tibial collateral ligament TCL (p. 47); abnormal mobility of the anterior drawer sign is due to anterior subluxation of the medial tibial condyle.

- The ADMR test is positive in extensive lesions affecting at least the anterior cruciate ligament ACL (p. 49) but generally not involving the fascia lata FL or the long fibular collateral ligament FCL-L[44]: the abnormal mobility of the anterior drawer sign is due to anterior subluxation of the medial tibial condyle.

The posterior drawer sign—rotation O; PDRO, the posterior drawer sign—lateral rotation PDLR, and the posterior drawer sign—medial rotation PDMR:

- Forced mobilization of the leg (see Figure 4.2), is obtained in a similar fashion, but backwards pressure is applied.

- The PDRO test is positive in specific lesion of the posterior cruciate ligament PCL (p. 49); the abnormal mobility of the drawer backwards sign is due to posterior subluxation of the tibial intercondylar space.

- The PDLR test is positive in extensive lesion affecting the lateral back corner LBC, the anterior horn of the lateral meniscus AFLM, the long fibular collateral ligament FCL-L, the posterior cruciate ligament PCL and the lateral posterior capsule LPC (p. 46); the abnormal mobility of the sign is due to posterior subluxation of the lateral tibial condyle.

- The PDMR test is positive in an extensive lesion affecting both the posterior cruciate ligament PCL and the medial posterior capsule MPC (p. 49); the abnormal mobility of the drawer backwards sign is due to posterior subluxation of the medial tibial condyle.

---

44 The anterior drawer sign—medial rotation ADMR—is usually very serious since it is present whenever there is very extensive capsuloligamentous lesion.

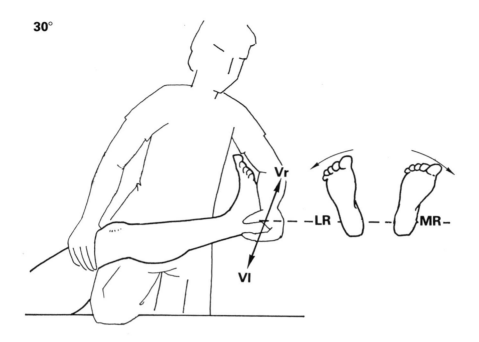

30°

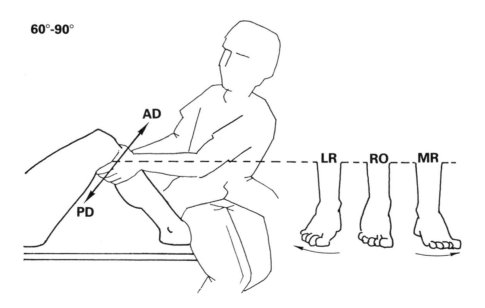

60°-90°

Dynamic pivot shift test PS

PS is pathognomonic of a lesion of the anterior cruciate ligament ACL. The abnormal medial rotation accompanied by a pivot shift, is due to anterior subluxation of the lateral tibial condyle followed by its reduction.

Biomechanical analysis.

The sector from 0° to 30° allows detection of any abnormal mobility in the 'mobile' lateral compartment (p. 37). In the 30° flexion position with medial rotation (p. 44) the lateral femoral condyle LFC is anchored by the ACL and rests against the anterior facet of the lateral tibial condyle LTC, near to its top T, which it is usually unable to cross (see Figure 4.22).

The slip occurs as extension is neared, with abnormal rearward movement of the lateral femoral condyle LFC, resulting in anterior subluxation ASL of the lateral tibial condyle LTC (see Figure 4.23).

The femoral condyle is freed from its moorings and is able to cross the intercondylar eminence, producing the slip before rolling onto the posterior facet of the tibial condyle. Subluxation of the tibial condyle is brought about by the quadriceps Q and the fascia lata FL (p. 56).

The recoil occurs at the initiation of flexion by reduction of the anterior subluxation of the lateral tibial condyle LTC (see Figure 4.24).

Reduction of subluxation of the joint surface occurs suddenly. At first it occurs passively, like a spring, due to elasticity and reflex muscle inhibition; and then actively due to the action of the biceps B and the fascia lata FL (p. 56) as active control of medial rotation is fairly rapidly regained[45]. The femoral condyle, freed from its moorings, is then able to cross the intercondylar eminence again, resulting in the jolt of reintegration, or recoil.

Signs and symptoms

Since the symptom of dislocation (p. 64) is a spontaneous demonstration of abnormal mobility, helped along by gravity, the PS test reproduces it as closely as possible through compression of the lateral compartment. This is obtained by opposing valgus-producing force to medial resistance; produced by passive mobilization of the leg which combines medial rotation and abduction; The medial resistance is provided by the medial meniscal, capsular and ligamentous apparatus and is

---

45 Previous tendinomuscular stretching accompanying anterior subluxation of the lateral tibial condyle makes it possible to anticipate a return to control of medial rotation, which occurs earlier than usual.

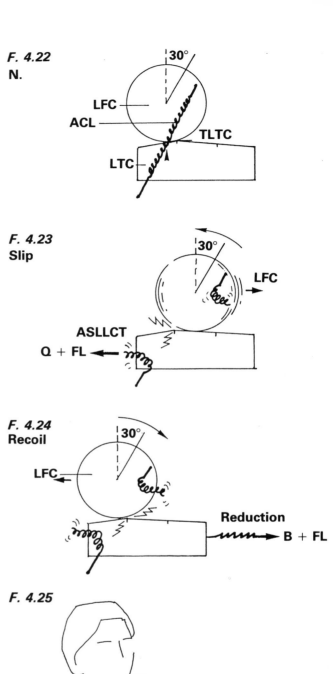

F. 4.22
N.

F. 4.23
Slip

F. 4.24
Recoil

F. 4.25

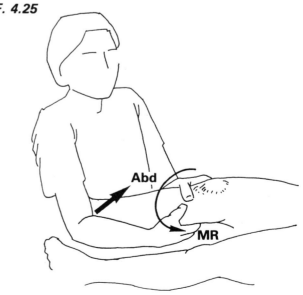

vigorous or weak depending on whether the apparatus is healthy or damaged.

Execution of the manoeuvre[46] by means of proximal, passive mobilization of the leg (see Figure 4.25), is facilitated by grasping the upper quarter with both hands. The patient's leg is held up by means of firmly gripping the foot between the examiner's elbow and chest, this leaves both hands free and the range of movement of the joint can be varied while medial rotation MR and abduction Abd are applied to the leg.

Additional findings

The patient is usually aware of the dislocation (p. 64) because of a sensation similar to that of the pivot shift. The painful rasping of the plane sign accompanies a somewhat vigorous response to the PS test. Maximum compression of the lateral femoral condyle nearly always succeeds in detecting any cartilaginous tibiofemoral lesion from the appearance of pain accompanying a grating sensation or sharp crunching.

In the presence of active or passive limitation of joint range of movement (pp. 68 and 70) in flexion, this investigation becomes virtually impossible.

Difficulties of interpretation are related to meniscal pathology. Transient impingement of a 'bucket handle' or of a posterior horn of the medial or lateral meniscus may resemble a vigorous pivot shift response by the lateral tibial condyle. Locking of the lateral tibial condyle in anterior subluxation, due to the impossibility of recoil, should not suggest meniscal locking since this type of locking occurs during flexion and unlocking is obtained immediately when the lateral compartment is decompressed.

Dynamic reverse pivot shift test RPS

The RPS test is pathognomonic for lesions of the posterolateral capsular and ligamentous structures. Abnormal lateral rotation, accompanied by a slip, is due to posterior subluxation of the lateral tibial condyle.

Biomechanical analysis

The sector of mobility extends from 30° to 60° and allows detection of abnormal mobility in the 'mobile' lateral compartment (p. 37). In 60° flexion position and with lateral rotation, (p. 45) the femoral condyle is seen resting on the anterior facet of the tibial condyle, after crossing the intercondylar eminence while sliding normally backward (see Figures 4.26 and 4.27). The slip occurs during flexion when the sudden posterior subluxation of the tibial condyle precipitates rearward movement

F. 4.26

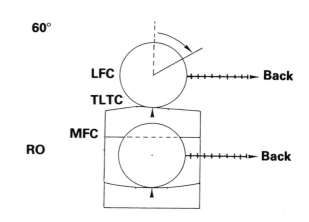

F. 4.27

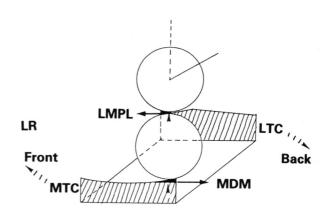

of the corresponding femoral condyle. The jerk as the eminence is crossed is part of a lateral rotation which is abnormal and disharmonious.

Signs and symptoms

The signs and symptoms are the same as for the pivot shift except that no recoil occurs.

---

46 The usual variants include the Lateral Pivot Shift test, J C Hughston's Jerk test, D Slocum's test, R E Losee's test, etc.

Laboratory tests

The ESR should be checked; a normal sedimentation rate is generally reassuring. Analyses of synovial fluid make it possible to establish three basic types[47].

The mechanical type, which is a pale straw-coloured and highly viscous fluid that does not clot spontaneously but has well formed mucin clots. It has low white cells (less than 5,000 per) and granulocyte counts (less than 25 per). Glucose and protein levels are normal, and bacteriological tests negative, but the fluid may contain calcium crystals.

The septic type, which is a grey, blood-streaked liquid with low viscosity which coagulates spontaneously but with no formation of mucin clots. It contains a high level of white cells (>100,000) and of granulocytes (>90), which are frequently defective. Glucose is low but protein is high. Bacteriological tests are positive but may be delayed or even produce false negative results.

The aseptic inflammatory type, which is intermediate between the other two. It resembles the mechanical type in moderate inflammation and is more like the septic type when there is definite inflammatory fluid.

X-ray examination

Standard X-ray examination

The X-ray examination must be comparative, routine and thorough. It must be routine because it is essential in orientating diagnosis and may be decisive in decisions involving indications of surgery; it must be comparative in order to detect minor modifications[48]; and it must be thorough and include at least five views.

Frontal view (Figure 4.28)

The standing patient's knees are fixed in extension with the feet placed parallel to one another, slightly apart. Any pelvispinal compensation must be

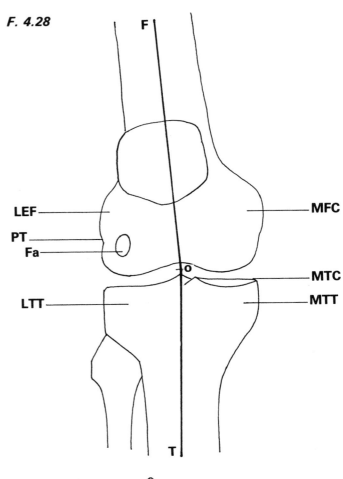

F. 4.28

FÔT # 174°

corrected (p. 66 and Note 28). In the normal conformation this position is that of the extended 'passive' knee (p. 33) with support by both legs (p. 61).

The lateral femoral condyle (p. 12) is noticeable because of the protrusion of the lateral epicondyle of the femur LEF (p. 18), the groove marking the insertion of the popliteal tendon PT and the fabella Fa (pp. 26 and Note 25) which may or may not project[49], but which has a characteristic coffee-bean shape. The medial femoral condyle (p. 12) is distinguished by the fact that it projects an area roughly similar to the lateral condyle although the protrusion of the medial femoral condyle is more sharply emphasized (p. 12). The patella is high and slightly laterally situated (p. 12) and is projected over the femoral condyles like a shield with the point reaching down at least as far as 1 cm above the joint interline.

---

47 Intra-articular injection of corticosteroids may change the nature of the fluid, notably by increasing capillary permeability, which may produce a misleadingly normal appearance for the synovial fluid.

48 The savings made by omitting comparative x-rays may be costly in terms of the harm that may occur by delay or uncertainty of diagnosis.

49 The fabella Fa becomes visible once it is ossified i.e. after adolescence.

The lateral tibial tuberosity LTT (p. 13) is superimposed over the medial half of the head of the fibula, with the tibiofibular joint space normally being somewhat open. The medial tibial tuberosity MTT (p. 13) is less prominent than the lateral LTT.

The joint interline is shaped like a flattened circumflex accent (or gable end) with roughly symmetrical sides. It can be identified after locating the outline of the medial tibial condyle MTC which is seen faintly superimposed as a concave form.

The tibiofemoral axis FOT equals 174° and corresponds to physiological valgum (p. 33).

Lateral view (see Figure 4.29)

The patient stands with the knee bent at a right angle with its lateral surface against the film. This position corresponds to the normal conformation in the 'passive' knee position in 90° flexion (p. 49) and has the advantage of giving a clear view of the patella and of both femoral condyles.

The patella is seen as a parallelipiped but with a somewhat convex anterior margin and a virtually straight posterior border, which lies behind the vertical line V that passes through the anterior tibial tuberosity ATT (p. 37).

The supratrochlear fossa appears empty and the junction with the upper margin of the trochlea is short and smooth.

The lateral tibiofemoral structures draw attention to a dense structure with regular outlines interrupted only by a notch corresponding to the intertrochlear crest of the lateral femoral condyle (p. 12). The lateral facet of the trochlea LFT and the notch are clearly distinguishable from the posterior margin of the patella, providing clear visibility of the patellofemoral interline. The lateral femoral condyle LFC can be distinguished; its posterior margin is particularly easy to identify since it is always aligned with the head of the fibula and sometimes with the fabella Fa.

The medial tibiofemoral structures are less dense[50] but also regular in outline. The medial facet of the trochlea MFT projects beyond the lateral facet and constitutes a sort of background to the tibiofemoral interline. The medial femoral condyle MFC also projects beyond its lateral tibial condyle, so that its posterior margin is superimposed over it. The anterior tibial tuberosity ATT is prominent.

---

50 The further the distance between these medial structures and the film the poorer the quality of the print.

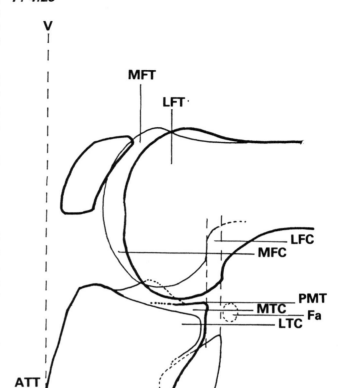

F. 4.29

The tibial condyles can be distinguished only at the rear: the overhanging outline of the medial through the intermediary of the posterior margin of the medial tibial condyle PMT (p. 13), is however more pronounced than that of the gentler slope of the lateral tibial condyle.

Tibiofemoral alignment can be assessed by drawing a vertical tangent at the posterior border of the medial femoral condyle MFC and of the lateral tibial condyle LTC. A variation in extension can be used to evaluate the tibiofemoral axis FOT at 180° against a vertical reference drawn at 0° extension (p. 33) and possibly at 190°, which provides physiological recurvatum of −10°.

The notch or tunnel view (see Figure 4.30)

The patient lies with the knee bent at a right angle. In terms of the standard conformation, this corresponds to the 'passive' knee, bent to 90° (p. 49) in order to reveal the bone structures which constitute the intercalary compartment (p. 38).

The intercondylar notch opens beneath the projected shadow of the patella and is like a regular, continuous arch. The femoral condyles reveal the posterior third of their articular surface and are curved around to the lateral facets of the notch. The lateral femoral condyle LFC can be identified from the presence of the groove of the popliteal tendon PT and the fibula in a lateral aspect. The intercondylar eminence IE of tibia is seen in its most favourable view.

Axial views of the patella (see Figures 4.31–4.33)

The patient lies down with the knee flexed at 30°, 60° and 90°. In terms of the standard conformation, this position corresponds to the 'passive' knee (p. 32) with the tibiofemoral joint viewed in successive longitudinal sections.

In the 30° axial view (see Figure 4.31), the position of the patella relative to the tibiofemoral joint can be established and the parameters of this joint can be determined. The patella is seen enclosed in the vertical line V which passes over the top of the lateral facet of the trochlea LFT. The crest of the patella fits the groove of the tibiofemoral joint.

In the 60° axial view (see Figure 4.32) the conformation of the patellofemoral joint (p. 12) can be examined and even measured. The patellar angle R is around 130°. The lateral facet of the patella LFP is at least as wide as the medial facet MFP. The angle of the trochlea T is around 140°. The lateral facet of the trochlea LFT is more prominent than the corresponding medial facet. The lateral patellofemoral interline and the medial patellofemoral interline are alike, apart from the slight inward deviation of the medial interline[51] due to tipping of the patella.

The 90° axial view (see Figure 4.33) reveals the onset of patellocondylar engagement and also shows the third articular facet of the patella F3P.

Additional Radiography

This is carried out only if required by the findings of the usual clinical radiological examination.

Plotting the anatomic and mechanical axes in extension

Plotting the axes in the frontal plane
The patient stands with the knees locked in extension with the feet parallel to each other and as

---

51 Apparent gaping of the medial femoropatellar space may also result in an error in the evaluation of the height of the lateral interline.

F. 4.30

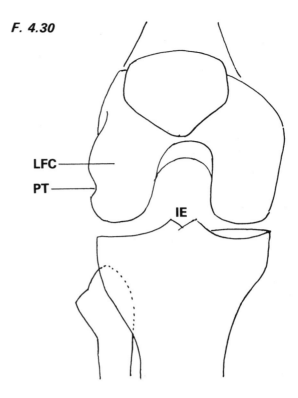

LFC
PT
IE

F. 4.31

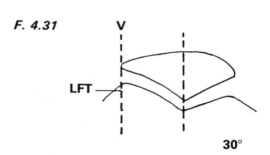

V
LFT
30°

F. 4.32

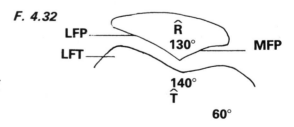

LFP
LFT
R̂
130°
MFP
140°
T̂
60°

F. 4.33

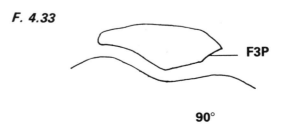

F3P
90°

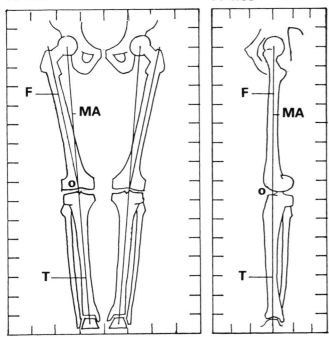

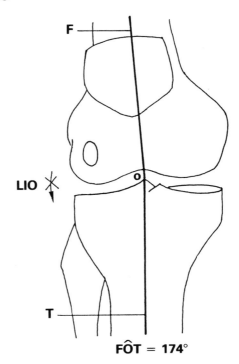

FÔT = 174°

close together as possible. The back is placed against the film and an opaque grid is used. In terms of the normal conformation, this corresponds to the extended 'active' knee (p. 53) with the weight on both feet.

The mechanical axis of the leg is visible on the frontal teleradiography (see Figure 4.34) as a straight line MA from the femoral head and the centre of the pulley of the talus, passing through the lateral tibial spine. The anatomic axes of femur and tibia are more clearly seen in the standard frontal view in extension (see Figure 4.36). The tibiofemoral angle FOT of 174° corresponds to physiological genu valgum (p. 77).

Plotting the axes in the sagittal plane
The patient stands with the knee screwed home in extension and its lateral surface against the film and an opaque grid is used. In terms of the normal conformation, this corresponds to the same conditions.

The mechanical axis of the leg is seen on the lateral teleradiography (see Figure 4.35) as a straight line MA from the femoral head to the centre of the pulley of the talus and passing through the pretibial space (p. 51 and Note 66). The anatomic axes of femur and tibia are more clearly seen in the standard lateral view in extension (see Figure 4.37) and form a tibiofemoral angle FOT of 180°, which equals 0° of extension, or, sometimes, to 190°, which equals −10° of physiologic genu recurvatum (p. 77).

F. 4.37

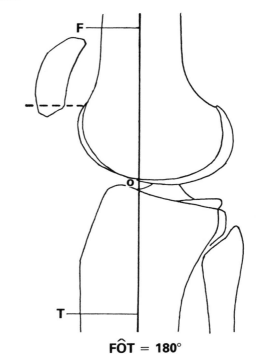

FÔT = 180°

The frontal view in extension

The patient stands with the knee locked in extension, with the back of the knee against the film. In terms of normal conformation (see Figure 4.36) this position corresponds to active balance with the weight on one leg (p. 61) so that the varus demands can be controlled without any opening of the lateral interline LIO.

The lateral view in extension

The patient stands with, and then without, voluntary contraction of the quadriceps, with the knee screwed home in extension with the lateral surface against the film. In terms of normal conformation, the patella (see Figure 4.37) is seen successively in a high position (p. 33) and then at maximum height (p. 53) while its lower edge may just reach the upper edge of the tibiofemoral joint, but is unable to go any higher.

F. 4.38

30°

60°

F. 4.39

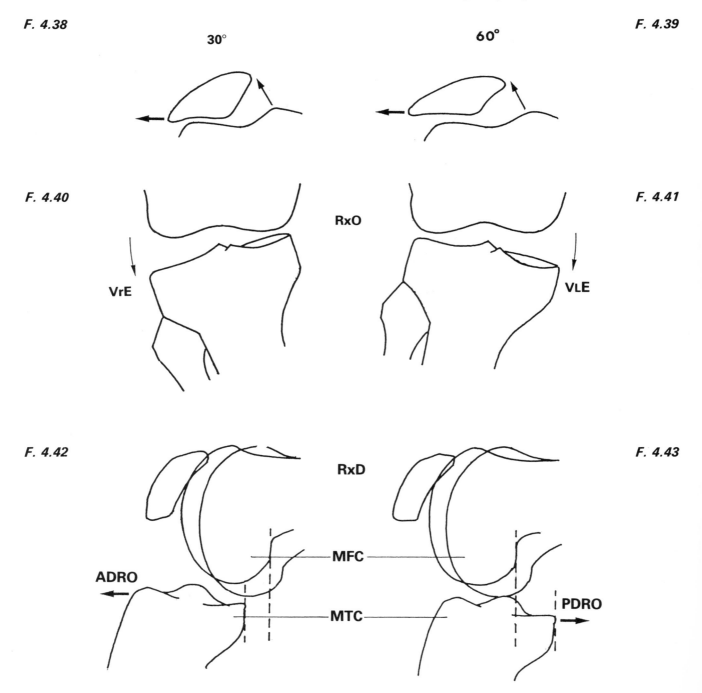

F. 4.40

RxO

VrE

VLE

F. 4.41

F. 4.42

RxD

ADRO

MFC

MTC

PDRO

F. 4.43

Reproduction of patellar imbalance (see Figures 4.38 and 4.39)

Contraction of the quadriceps and lateral rotation are combined with 30° and 60° axial views of the patella.

Voluntary reproduction of lateral subluxation or dislocation of the patella may involve lateral displacement of the patella as a result of force from the quadriceps, and this is amplified because of the lateral rotation[52]. However, the usefulness of this manoeuvre is limited because of the contradictory results obtained; in some patients, this reproduction of imbalance may result in either a shift away from the centre or towards the centre.

Reproduction of the lateral opening or radiodynamic opening or RxO (see Figures 4.40 and 4.41).

Passive mobilization of the leg with abduction or adduction (p. 70) is combined with a frontal view carried out in full extension with the patient lying down (p. 76). Visualization of opening of the lateral or medial interline can provide confirmation of valgus extension VlE or varus extension VrE.

Reproduction of the drawer sign—rotation O or radiodynamic drawer sign RxD (see Figures 4.42 and 4.43).

Passive mobilization of the leg with the application of forwards or backwards pressure in rotation O (p. 72) is combined with a lateral view in 90° of flexion (p. 77) and has the advantage of providing a reference for comparison. Forced reproduction of the abnormal mobility is seen as the loss of vertical alignment of the back of the medial femoral condyle MFC with that of the medial tibial condyle MTC. Visualization of anterior or posterior subluxation of the tibia confirms the clinical observation of the anterior drawer sign—rotation O ADRO or of the posterior drawer sign—rotation O PDRO[53].

Special tests

Aspiration

Aspiration of effusion makes it easier to carry out identification and measurements and reduces the defence reaction (p. 68), which increases the precision of clinical and radiological examination.

Depending on the appearance of the fluid:

- Haemarthrosis is merely aspirated and is indicative of severity.

- Pyarthrosis, hydrohaemarthrosis and hydrarthrosis are aspirated and the fluid withdrawn is subjected to laboratory tests (p. 76).

Arthrography

Interarticular examination with contrast media may involve positive contrast media, gas or both (double contrast): each technique has its supporters and its critics. Positive contrast is the preferred technique at present for reasons of practicability, low cost, and the data it provides.

Its practicability is related above all to the patient; it is painless and brief, and comfortable examinations are readily accepted. Its painlessness particularly depends on the skill with which the intra-articular injection is administered. This demands careful insertion of the needle, which should not be felt; filling of the joint cavity by a volume of contrast medium equal to its capacity, but without exceeding the threshold of pain related to distension[54]; uniform dispersal of the contrast medium, simply by means of active and passive movement; manoeuvres intended to widen the joint spaces are painful and can be eliminated.

Speed is essential in the radiographs, since they must be completed within five minutes[55].

---

52 The alignment of the extensor apparatus in the frontal plane should usually begin at 30° of flexion (p. 41) and be fully achieved at 60° (p. 45): lateral rotation operates against this alignment and produces the smallest QRT angle possible by means of the most powerful lateral displacement force possible; this force may be responsible for subluxation or dislocation.

53 The bony disc of the disinsertion of a posterior or anterior cruciate ligament from the floor, follows the femur during its displacements relative to the tibia.

54 The volume of the joint varies between 10 ml and 50 ml. It should be filled until resistance to injection is encountered and reflux begins to occur.

55 The outline provided by the positive contrast medium has the unfortunate drawback of rapid loss of clarity and definition.

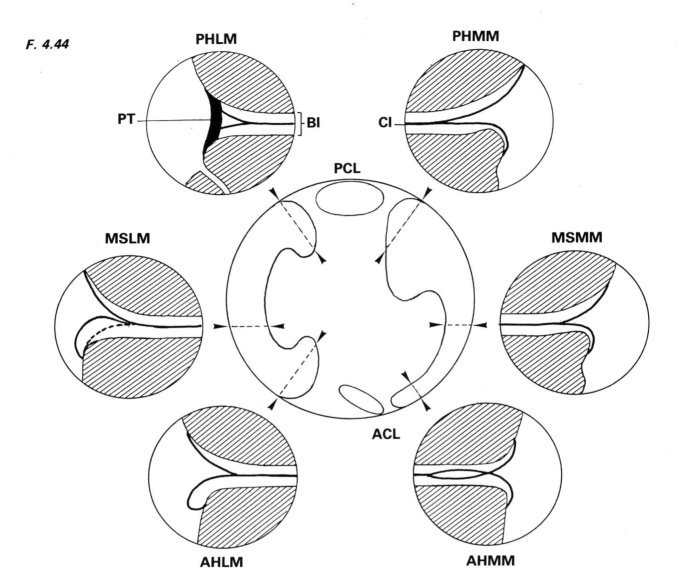

F. 4.44

PHLM

PHMM

PT — ⎬ BI

CI

PCL

MSLM

MSMM

ACL

AHLM

AHMM

Comfort is obtained largely as a result of the previous aspiration of the effusion and the subsequent aspiration of the contrast medium as soon as the examination has been completed.

The cost is low because only about ten plates are required, since both menisci are viewed simultaneously in a given view.

The data obtained is relatively exhaustive and more complete than that obtained by simple meniscography[56] because of the number of positions, in terms of the standard conformation which can be obtained.

Circular views, carried out in full extension, explore the tibiofemoral joint through 180° during several rotations (see Figure 4.44). The menisci are seen in sagittal section which passes through the horns and the middle segment to provide a normal angular image[57] which varies slightly depending on whether they are lateral or medial. The large posterior horn of the medial meniscus PHMM contrasts with the slightly smaller anterior horn of the lateral mensicus AHLM. The middle segment of the medial meniscus MSMM can be distinguished from the corresponding lateral structure MSLM, which is often masked by a false submeniscal recess[58]. The

56 The opaque liquid clearly defines all the contours of the joint space by spreading regularly over the surface of the menisci and of the cartilaginous covering, the notch and the fully distended capsule.

57 The normal meniscus shows regular transparency and an acutely angular outline, the top and sides of which correspond to the free edge and the upper and lower surfaces.

58 This false submeniscal recess results from the interposition of the convex lateral plateau tibia (p. 12).

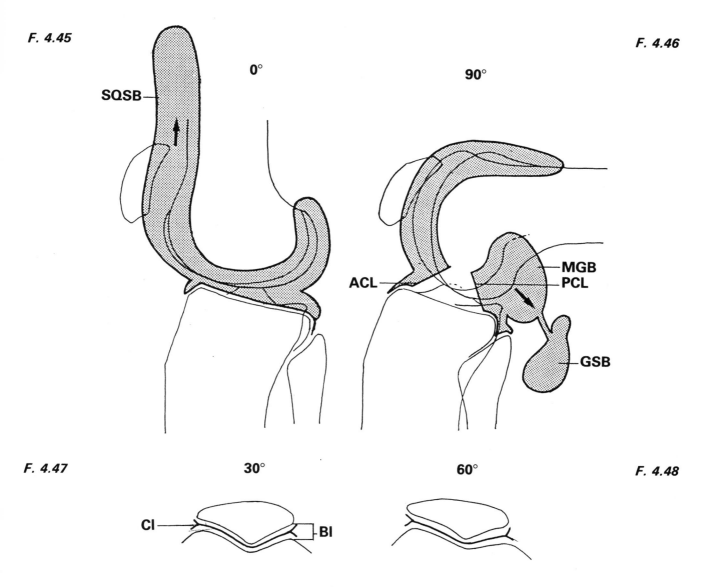

F. 4.45

SQSB

0°

F. 4.45

SQSB

0°

90°   **F. 4.46**

ACL

MGB
PCL

GSB

F. 4.47   **30°**   **60°**   **F. 4.48**

CI → BI

slender anterior horn of the medial meniscus AHMM contrasts with the bulkier posterior horn of the lateral meniscus PHLM, which is bordered vertically and peripherally by the normal opacity of the popliteal tendon PT.

The capsule, which is invisible, is continuous in front of the meniscofemoral and meniscotibial spaces, and is inseparable from the wall of the meniscus. The cartilage interline CI is visible as a fringe some distance from the edges of the bone interline BI.

Lateral views in extension[59] (see Figure 4.45) and flexion[60] (see Figure 4.46). The subquadricipital serous bursa SqSB (p. 14) balloons out and is regular and clearly delimited. The medial gastrocnemius bursa MGB (p. 20) and sometimes the gastrocnemio-semimembranosus bursa GSB

(p. 26) communicate via a narrow channel[61]. The MGB is ovoid in shape and the GSB long and thin; both are regularly and clearly outlined. The cruciate ligaments can be detected, the ACL within its sheath, from its anterior margin, and the PCL by its posterior edge.

Axial 30° and 60° views of the patella (and sometimes the 90° axial view) (see Figures 4.47 and 4.48). The cartilaginous interline CI normally appears as a border at some distance from the bone interline,

59 Extension aids filling of the anterior portion of the joint cavity.

60 Flexion drives the contrast medium out of the posterior portion of the joint cavity and opens the connecting channel between the two bursae.

61 This channel may sometimes be visible as it emerges from the middle of the posterior surface of the medial gastrocnemius bursa and slopes downwards and backwards towards the closed gastrocnemio-semimembranosus bursa.

83

with two-pronged ends. The capsule is invisible and continuous in front of the synovial alar folds but cannot be distinguished from the patellar retinacula (pp. 18 and 20).

Overall, contrast arthrography should be revived in view of the wealth of data provided at the 'lowest cost'. However, its usefulness is tempered by two factors: the success of the positive contrast method depends to a greater extent on the skill of the operator rather than on the medium used; and the positive contrast method is highly successful in the domain of exploration of the lateral compartments of the tibiofemoral joint, particularly of the posterior third, but is ineffective when used to investigate the central pivot.

Arthroscopy

Arthroscopy is currently gaining importance in diagnosis and simplification of treatment. It is especially suitable for some rheumatological conditions, especially incipient rheumatoid arthritis, which can be distinguished from isolated synovitis by means of biopsy taken under visual monitoring and treated by means of synovial orthosis.

Though it is not for routine use, arthroscopy is of major interest in traumatology as a complementary examination, and preferable to arthrography, for exploring the cartilaginous covering of the lateral and intercalary compartments.

Routine use of the technique is hindered by both technical and practical considerations. The exploration may be misleading as a result of partial intrasynovial rupture of the anterior cruciate ligament ACL (p. 17 and Note 13), or inconclusive in the posterior portion of medial compartment, where arthrography is particularly successful.

It is possible to envisage its use in the extraction of a foreign body, but it does not repair disinsertion of the meniscus or a capsular and ligamentous lesion.

The practical aspects are the same as for any surgery and this imposes a need for rigorous asepsis, general or epidural anaesthesia, the use of a pneumatic tourniquet, etc. Because the technique borders on surgery, arthrography is always to be preferred if the findings of the clinical examination justify this.

Tomography

Indications for sagittal or frontal sections are unusual in the field of joint trauma and are justified only to elucidate an indecisive standard plate.

CAT SCAN

Sequential horizontal sections of the leg seen by computerised axial tomography provide accurate information about the details of the various bony parts and the articulations which connect them. The patient lies down, but the legs are in a position as near as possible to that during walking i.e. in the stepping angle (p. 66 and Note 25).

The standard conformation of images is a series of sections from top to bottom establishing the following features.

Anteposition AP or retroposition RP of the femoral head (see Figure 4.49) with regard to the posterior margin of the pelvis Pv, which represents the frontal plane.

The medial femoral angle of torsion represented by the angle of anteversion of the neck of the femur POC (see Figure 4.50) between the longitudinal axis of the neck and the transverse axis through the two femoral condlyes C^{62}, equal to about $15°$[63].

The position of the patella relative to the tibiofemoral joint and the patellofemoral conformation (see Figure 4.50), in terms of the norms already described (p. 78), which here have the advantage of being applied between $0°$ and $30°$ i.e. in the sector at the onset of mobility which is the most frequently involved, but which escapes standard examination.

The distance d (see Figure 4.51) between the anterior tibial tuberosity ATT and the throat of the trochlea TT, which gives an indication of the position of the tibia beneath the femur during lateral rotation (p. 33).

The tibiofemoral angle of divergence COT (see Figure 4.51) between the transverse axis through the two femoral condyles C^{62} and the transverse axis through the two tuberosities T^{64}, which theoretically establishes the position of the tibia beneath the femur during approximately $5°$ lateral rotation (p. 33).

The angles of lateral tibial torsion[65], which are ● the angle COM (see Figure 4.52) between the transverse axis of the two condyles C^{62} and the

---

62 The tangent to the posterior outline of the lateral and medial condyles of femur corresponds to a precisely plotted line.

63 The marked anteversion of the neck of the femur at birth rapidly decreases from $40°$ to $15°$ and is fixed by the end of growth.

64 The tangent to the posterior outline of the lateral and medial tibial tuberosities may often be a variable line because of the correspondence of the slope to that of the lateral joint surface of tibia (p. 12).

65 The low degree of lateral tibial torsion at birth very quickly increases from $2°$ to $20°$ and is fixed by the end of infancy.

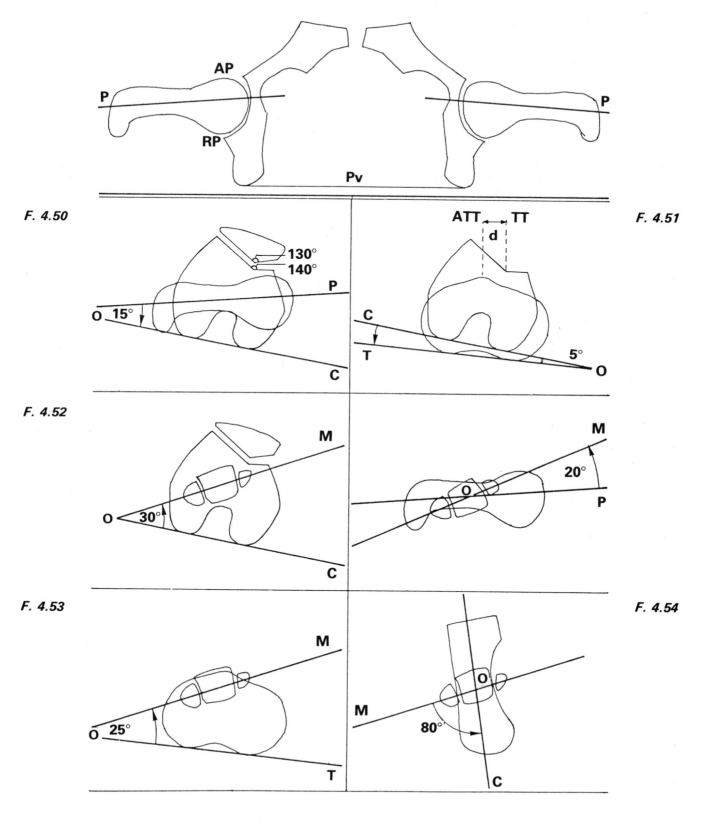

F. 4.49

F. 4.50

F. 4.51

F. 4.52

F. 4.53

F. 4.54

bimalleolar axis M, which equals at approximately 30°. ● the angle TOM (see Figure 4.53) between the transverse axis of the two tuberosities T[64] and the bimalleolar transverse axis M, which is less reliably evaluated at approximately 25°.

The talocalcaneal angle of divergence[66], which is the same as the angle MOC (see Figure 4.54) between the bimalleolar transverse axis M and the longitudinal axis of the calcaneus C, which is equal to approximately 80°.

The angle of torsion of the leg POM (see Figure 4.56) between the longitudinal axis of the projection of the neck of the femur P and the bimalleolar transverse axis M, which is equal to approximately 20°[67].

Examination under general anaesthesia

Passive tests for abnormal mobility (p. 70 et seq) may be significant only under general anaesthesia which should, theoretically, provide optimum examination conditions for the passive knee during muscle relaxation and elimination of any defence reaction (p. 68).

Scintigraphic osteoarticular exploration

Selective fixation of the tracer by the bone makes it possible to investigate the topography and level of reactional osteogenesis which occurs in response to any aggression[68], with the added advantage of being feasible before radiological signs develop. The detection of a focus or zone of abnormal hyperactivity should be confirmed in a lateral view[69] and by comparative examination.

Exploration of the soft tissues

Xeroradiography

Detailed analysis on a single film of the superficial, aponeurotic, tendinomuscular and osseous levels is facilitated by the 'interface effect': the boundaries between structures of differing densities are clearly differentiated to the point of giving an apparent three-dimensional effect.

Thermography

Determination of the infra red rays emitted from the surface provides topographic and quantitative information concerning and the vascular or neurovascular involvement in an inflammatory reaction[70]. The detection of an abnormally hot or cold area (in comparision with the reference thermograph) should be checked by comparative examination.

Ultrasound

In ultrasound, the anatomic display includes the surface, aponeurotic and especially tendinomuscular levels (the latter has uniform ultrasound-reflecting structures[71]: any area which is exceptionally reflective, transparent, patchy or that combines these features, should be checked and the findings compared with those obtained using thermography, although complete agreement cannot always be expected.[72].

---

66 The divergence between the talus and the calcaneus decreases as the talus straddles the calcaneus; the foot is flat at birth but should normally become arched. This occurs gradually due to the riding up of the tarsus followed by the rising of the instep.

67 The cervico-bimalleolar index is consequently formed by medial torsion of the femur and lateral torsion of the tibia.

68 The basic scintigraphic image of fresh bone tissue can be processed 'geographically' into isoactive curves.

69 The lateral incidence can, if the tracer has been evenly distributed, identify the site of osseous hyperactivity with certainty as patellar, femoral or tibial.

70 The thermographic image obtained can be processed by a computer to provide isotherms.

71 The bone level is not visible since the bone cortex constitutes a barrier to ultrasound.

72 Echography and thermography can be considered complementary in the examination of various tendinomuscular lesions.

Chapter 5
PATHOLOGY

Articular and periarticular traumatology account for an essential part of the pathology we are considering here. Also, polymicrotraumatology and the new ground it covers is taken into account. This includes conditions caused by the excessive constraints that occur mostly in sports and occasionally in certain occupations (p. 53 and Note 71), and which are based on performing a normal movement or being in a normal position but with abnormal demands in terms of intensity, duration, frequency or coordination.

The population covered in this section ranges from the child to the young adult, and includes the critical period of adolescence.

Bone pathology and joint pathology, e.g. fractures and bone infections, tumours and arthritis do not come within the scope of this account.

Isolated meniscal lesions

The particular vulnerability of the menisci is caused partially by the fact that they are composite structures, consisting of tendon, capsule and ligament tissue, as well as cartilaginous tissue (p. 15 and Note 11).

Classic lesion of the medial meniscus

Since the isolated lesion of the medial meniscus normally flagrantly indicates its presence, it is the best known and consequently the most frequently diagnosed.

Pathogenesis

The pathogenesis is stereotyped. The site of involvement is elective, nearly always including the posterior horn and middle segment, but not the anterior horn (p. 46 and Note 49).

The traumatic nature[1] is significant in the presence of a tear or a disinsertion, whose simultaneously

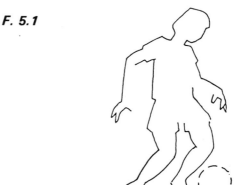

F. 5.1

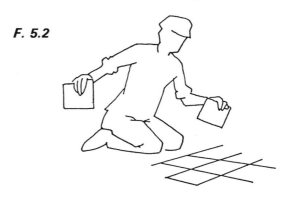

F. 5.2

vertical and longitudinal components will establish a gap between the upper and lower stages of the meniscus. The trigger mechanism involves single foot support (Figure 5.1) in valgus-flexion/lateral rotation[2], or two-foot support (Figure 5.2) in a hyperflexed position[3]. The lesion begins at the junction of the posterior horn and the middle segment (Figure 5.3) and spreads rearward or forward. The tear follows the crescent-shaped alignment of the longitudinal fibres and breaks the fibrocartilage into fragments. A number of conditions can result, including the bucket-handle tear with intrusion into the intercondylar notch.

Disinsertion[4] frees the fibrocartilage, which remains intact but capable of luxation[5].

---

1 The traumatic lesion of the medial meniscus is more frequent than malformation and degeneration; in fact, malformation is more common in the lateral meniscus, while degeneration of the medial meniscus is usually secondary to disalignment of the tibiofemoral axis in varum.

2 Overloading single foot support (p. 51) in combination with rotation creates a situation that has both vertical and longitudinal components.

3 Kneeling and sitting on the heels, positions used by tile or carpet layers, enables the meniscus to become disattached and undergo luxation. Disattachment of the meniscus from the posterolateral capsule is caused by excessive constraints in complete flexion (p. 49). Intra-articular meniscal luxation is produced during kneeling because the normal posterior recall function is not in operation since the semimembranous muscle is relaxed (p. 30), and the situation is more critical during rising because the normal anterior recall function of the medial meniscopatellar ligament (p. 35) is operating.

4 Rupture of the meniscocapsulary attachments occurs along the border area corresponding to the capsule on one side and the meniscal wall on the other (pp. 15 and 16).

5 Luxation may occur during an operation, the meniscus hook easily pulling the posterior horn in front of the condyle.

Clinical examination

The clinical examination can be expected to provide sufficient data for diagnosis of typical cases. The interview is descriptive with the memory of an 'acute accident' linked to sudden locking. The determining feature of the examination involves locking in extension (pp. 64, 66 and 70) with the sensation of an elastic limit peculiar to meniscal luxation[6].

Special examinations

They serve no purpose except in atypical cases. Opaque arthrography (p. 81) always makes it possible to differentiate between a tear and a disinsertion, with the latter capable of responding to meniscal reinsertion as the indication of choice[7]. Arthroscopy (p. 84) is not easy to use in exploration of the posterior part of the medial compartment.

Course (Figures 5.4–5.9)

This course cannot be predicted because it is based on four possibilities:

- The appearance of locking indicates the extension of the intial lesion.
- The persistence of locking requires arthrotomy.
- Progressive decrease of locking through enlargement of the opening.
- Sudden reduction of locking, spontaneous or manual, accompanied by an instantaneous and audible return.

F. 5.3

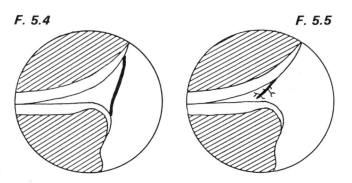

F. 5.4   *F. 5.5*

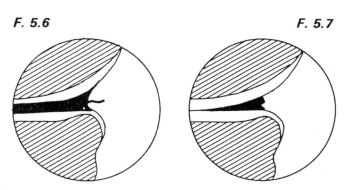

F. 5.6   *F. 5.7*

F. 5.8   *F. 5.9*

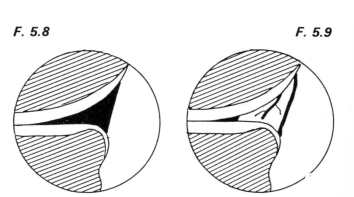

---

6 Since locking in complete extension is not always apparent, the examination can be refined by using the 'at attention' position (p. 61), with inspection being carried out with lateral view and the knee against a hard vertical surface; the injured knee remains stiff in its incorrect position at some distance from the reference surface, and any attempt at alignment is blocked.

7 There are a number of possible modifications of the normal arthrographic image (p. 82 and Note 57): disinsertion with a vertical line transforming the acute angle into a triangle (Figure 5.4);

- the tear with an oblique line 'breaking' the uniformity (Figure 5.5);
- degeneration with a horizontal line extending the thickening of the cartilaginous interline (Figure 5.6);
- partial luxation of a strip separating from the meniscal wall (Figure 5.7);
- complete luxation creating a meniscal 'empty area' (Figure 5.8);
- combined disinsertion-tearing-degeneration-partial luxation etc., producing a number of variations (Figure 5.9).

Lesion of the lateral meniscus

In principal, the isolated lesion of the lateral meniscus is as frequent as that of the medial meniscus. It has its particular characteristics.

Pathogenesis

Classification is impossible because the site of involvement is not elective; the lesion can spread to the entire meniscus or be limited to either the anterior or the posterior horns, or the middle segment. The three types of lesion can be classified as trauma, malformation and degeneration.

The traumatic lesion[8] has a vertical tear, leaving a gap between the upper and lower meniscal stages. There are 3 types.

1) Longitudinal type (Figure 5.10) where the tear and disinsertion follow the crescent-shaped path of the horizontal fibrocartilaginous fibres (Figure 2.15). The trigger mechanism is based on single foot support in varus-flexion/medial rotation (Figure 3.46) or two-footed support in hyperflexion (Figure 5.2).

The lesion may begin in the middle segment[9] and spreads forward and rearward, culminating in a bucket handle capable of luxation and in disinsertion that proceeds by enlarging the popliteal hiatus PH.

2) The transverse type (Figure 5.11) is specific to the lateral meniscus. The tear starts at the free border and continues toward the peripheral surface. The trigger mechanism is based on sudden compression of the lateral compartment, with forced axial movement of the knee in flexion, or forced lateral movement with direct impact on the knee in extension. The lesion begins in the middle segment[10], and culminates by dividing the meniscus into anterior and posterior halves.

3) The oblique type (Figure 5.12) is intermediary between the two preceding lesions, the 'aborted' tear starting on the free border and continuing some distance before turning parallel to the peripheral surface. The trigger mechanism essentially involves forced rotation. The lesion begins in the middle segment and produces a 'strip'.

---

8 The so-called conventional post-traumatic lesion implies an initial accident as the cause.

9 The large amount of mobility of the lateral meniscus explains the vulnerability of the middle segment, which is more highly exposed to laceration or detachment during back and forth longitudinal movement.

10 The condyle can crush the middle segment on the chopping block of the convex area of the tibial condyle.

F. 5.10

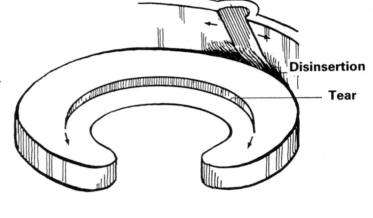

PH

Disinsertion

Tear

F. 5.11

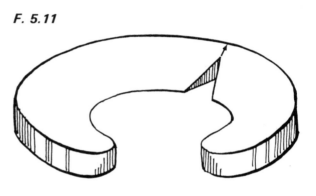

F. 5.12

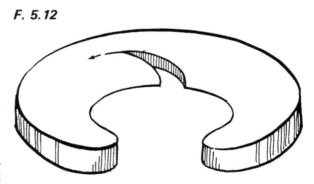

The malformation called the 'disc-shaped' meniscus[11] summarizes a multiplicity of anomalous shapes and insertions.

1) The anomaly of shape is varied and can be any of the following.

The single complete meniscus, usually thinner in the centre, but totally separating the upper and lower stages of the meniscus (Figure 5.13).

The doughnut-shaped meniscus that makes a nearly complete circle around a central opening that provides for communication between the two stages (Figure 5.14).

The two-level meniscus with a horizontal split from the anterior horn to the posterior horn (Figure 5.15).

The comma-shaped, crown-shaped and O-shaped menisci, as well as those that are disc-shaped in the strictest sense, with median relief, etc.

2) Insertion anomalies are also varied, anterior, median or posterior, with the corresponding meniscal segment being unattached and capable of luxation.

The degenerative lesion[12] is illustrated by horizontal cracks on the upper or lower facet, but without a break in continuity between the upper and lower meniscal stages (Figure 5.16).

1) The longitudinal type is typical and representative, with cracks following the crescent-shaped path of the horizontal fibres on one of the two fibrocartilaginous surfaces. The mechanism is based on polymicrotraumatology (p. 87). The lesion is distributed on the basis of the number and length of the cracks.

2) Meniscal calcification and meniscal lamination[13] occur atypically.

On the whole, the pathogenesis of the isolated lesion of the lateral meniscus is more often complex than straightforward, defying any classification as soon as associations and the course enter the picture.

F. 5.13

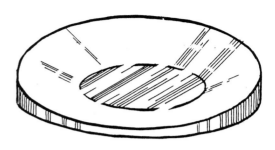

F. 5.14

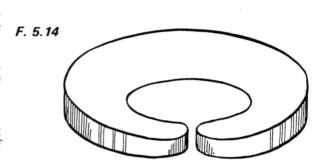

F. 5.15

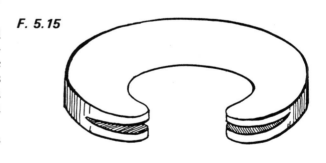

F. 5.16

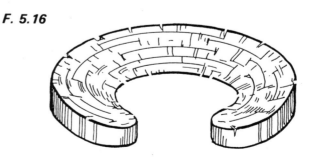

---

11 This constitutional anomaly is of unknown origin and probably, but not necessarily, congenital: in fact, characteristic horizontal partitioning in the 'disc-shaped' stage of meniscal embryogenesis cannot be confirmed.

12 Equivalent to 'wearing' with microscopic and macroscopic modifications.

13 Small surface streaks or microcracks suggest a lesion caused by hammering or shearing.

Associated conditions make it impossible to demonstrate the initial site of involvement[14] with the possible exception of the vertical tear, which can be considered isolated only in specific transverse tears of the lateral meniscus. The course makes it impossible to recognize the initial nature of the condition[15], with the exception of the peripheral cyst, which has a common outcome.

In fact, cyst formation[16] may modify the lateral meniscus in any lesion that begins with a notch or slot and terminates in a cyst.

No matter how it begins, a lesion is predisposed to form a cyst if the breach is horizontal. This can be caused by the following:

● Trauma when a vertical tear, longitudinal, transverse or oblique, is combined with a horizontal slit.

● Malformation where a horizontally split two-level meniscus exists.

● Degeneration where there are horizontal cracks.

The slot can result from centrifugal spread of the lesion in the horizontal plane. When it arises on one of the meniscal facets, the tibial or femoral[17], the slot is both horizontal and recessed (Figure 5.17). The end closest to the intercondylar notch communicates with the joint cavity as soon as the horizontal breach occurs; the end furthest from the intercondylar notch reflects the horizontal progress of 'transmeniscal drilling' leading to the formation of a cyst above the capsular surface (Figures 5.18–5.21).

Since it is subjected to tangential force in the horizontal plane (Figure 5.23), the slot can only spread away from the centre of the joint[18]; the centrifugal liquid current drives joint fluid into the slot[19], preventing spontaneous healing.

The cyst erupts on the exterior of the anterior horn or at the junction between the anterior horn and the middle segment. Histodiagnosis[20] makes it possible to verify a cyst cavity because it is always linked to the joint cavity in macroscopic as well as microscopic appearance. *Macroscopically* in that the cavitation is more voluminous and unilocular, being intermittently perceptible; *microscopically* in that the cavitation is more diffuse and multilocular, remaining unapparent.

Clinical examination

The clinical examination may offer no convincing diagnosis.

The interview is summarized by an indication of isolated lateral difficulty, compatible with daily activities and sometimes with the requirements of the occupation or sport pursued.

The examination may be decisive if a meniscal cyst is found erupting under the fascia lata at the anterolateral part of the interline. The cyst is normally painful before becoming visible and palpable, but pain is sometimes only intermittent, occurring during a 'subacute attack'. A painful premonitory symptom may be the only manifestation: a 'horizontal' shooting pain from the lateral interline, with a mechanical pattern that subsequently becomes mixed making it necessary to utilize a particular position that forces the interline open for relief of pain. Symptoms are often evident: the rounded or ovoid swelling is highly visible in extension, but disappears rearward under the fascia lata in complete flexion. Palpation is always demonstrative but particularly at the initiation of flexion, when the fascia lata tenses and consequently inhibits rearward movement of the cyst. Painful swelling offers resistance to the finger and sometimes a hardening occurs that may simulate a 'second head of the fibula' at maximum size.

Exteriorization is intermittent: during a cyclic course, reduction may be instantaneous in forced or gradual varus movement, so that the inflammatory crisis is replaced with calm obtained through rest.

Special examinations

Special examinations are most often necessary.

---

14 Segmental lesions (anterior horn—middle segment—posterior horn) and complete lesions (example: complete bucket handle or whole meniscus) offer a large number of possible combinations.

15 The three entities (trauma, malformation and degeneration) are linked by transitional forms, including the traumatic lesion modified by secondary degeneration, the lesion on top of malformation modified and revealed by trauma or by secondary degeneration.

16 Cyst-formation can be described by other terms including cyst or pseudocyst, mucoid or myxoid degeneration, etc.

17 The meniscal slot does not break the continuity between the upper and lower meniscal stages.

18 Tangential force is reflected in the lateral constraints whose resultant LC is orientated outward (p. 61 and Note 99).

19 The composition of the cyst fluid is similar to that of synovial fluid.

20 Anatopathological comparisons are always significant. The *cyst* dissociates and modifies the crescent-shaped horizontal fibres on either the superior or inferior surfaces. The *cyst cavity* does not have its own wall or may be synovialized, but is always linked to the joint cavity through a fistular channel. The *meniscal wall* reacts by capsular hyperplasia and synovialization. The fibrocartilage shows the horizontal breach resulting from a lesion that may be the result of trauma, malformation or degeneration.

F. 5.17

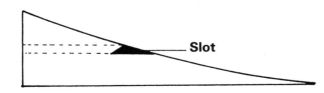

Slot

Opaque arthrography (p. 81) may provide positive diagnosis on the basis of an atypical clinical form, up to the point of specifying the pathogenetic variation and course through its highly detailed images: this means that the cyst of the lateral meniscus can be seen in totality when the contrast medium outlines the horizontal slot before filling the cyst cavity (Figure 5.22) (p. 91).

Arthroscopy (p. 84) may make up for any insufficiency of opaque arthrography by offering as diversified a picture with the exception of the cyst, of which only the entry orifice can be seen.

Course

The course is subacute with crises, leading sooner or later to arthrotomy.

F. 5.18

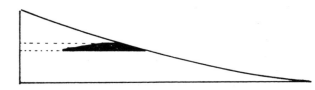

F. 5.19

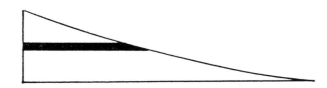

F. 5.20

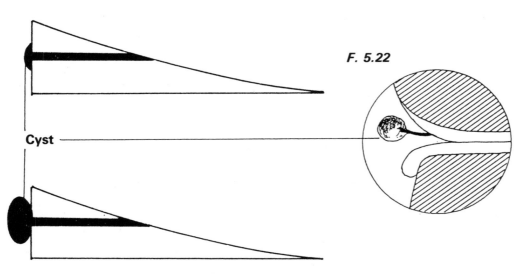

F. 5.22

Cyst

F. 5.21

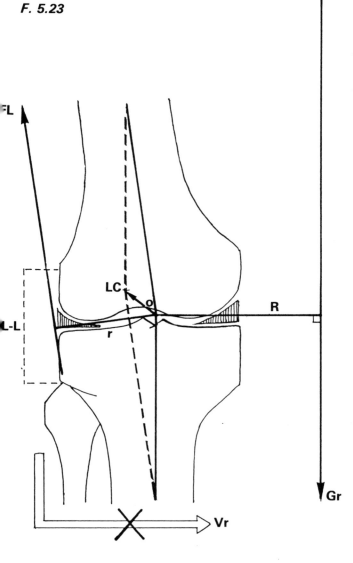

FL x r = Gr x R

Meniscal, Capsular and Ligamentous Lesion

Meniscal, capsular and ligamentous lesions are the characteristics of the basic sprain (p. 63 and Note 7). There are two forms, that are defined on the basis of the initial accident: acute or recent lesion manifested during the first ten days, and the chronic or delayed lesion.

Acute or recent form

When a lesion manifests itself within ten days after the initial accident, the primary consideration is to decide whether it is serious or benign.

Serious lesion with tear or disinsertion (p. 63 and Note 4)

This lesion is diagnosed in terms of its severity, in order to determine the orthopaedic or surgical treatment of choice[21]. Presumptive indications of seriousness can be ranked in chronological order.

The three signs of alarm at the time of the initial accident are 'syncopal' pain, snapping, immediate and total incapacity (p. 63). There is also haemarthrosis determined by aspiration (p. 81) or ecchymosis, which is usually delayed and lopsided. There is persistent incapacity through locking or dislocation.

Signs are best determined during clinical and x-ray examinations to be carried out under the best conditions[22]. The signs are:

- True locking (pp. 64, 66 and 70; Note 14).
- Abnormal movements (p. 68 et seq).
- The bone fragment characteristic of a disinsertion.
- Radiodynamic opening RxO or radiodynamic drawer sign RxD (p. 81).

Benign lesion occurring in distension

This assumption is made once a diagnosis of a serious lesion has been eliminated, and before undertaking medical or physical treatment.

---

21 The lesion inventory is 'accessory' in relation to the urgent need to establish the seriousness of the lesion within the first ten days, the period of time in which the lesion is in fresh condition, and consequently presents the most propitious conditions for immediate reconstruction.

22 The best examination conditions occur under two sets of circumstances: *possibly* in the field when complete reflex muscular incapacity occurs at the time of the accident; *preferably* in an operating theatre with the facilities for aspiration and the use of general anaesthesia.

Chronic or delayed form

The serious lesion which does not receive appropriate treatment in the first ten days after the initial accident should be considered as having become chronic.

Classification of chronic lesions

Knee position in the initial accident is used as the basis for distinguishing between ligamentous injury occurring during flexion and that occurring during extension.

Ligamentous injury occurring during flexion is also called rotary injury[23], and consists of six conditions that are divided into three groups on the basis of the direction of rotation:

- Isolated lesion of the anterior cruciate ligament variation 1, anterolateral laxity and posteromedial laxity variation 1 corresponding to medial rotary ligamentous injury.

- Anteromedial laxity + posterolateral laxity variation 1 corresponding to a lateral rotary ligamentous injury.

- Isolated lesion of the posterior cruciate ligament corresponding to a ligamentous injury in rotation O.

Ligamentous injury in extension[24] consists of six conditions that are divided into three groups on the basis of similarity:

- Isolated lesion of the anterior cruciate ligament variation 2 + posterior laxity.

- Posterolateral laxity variation 2 + antero-posteriolateral laxity.

- Posteromedial laxity variation 2 + antero-posteriomedial laxity.

F. 5.24

F. 5.25

F. 5.26

ACL

MR

ASL LTC

---

23 The flexed knee is relatively less vulnerable; in fact excess biomechanical energy is largely absorbed by being shunted into rotation.

24 The stretched knee position is relatively more vulnerable: in fact, excess biomechanical energy has no possibility of being shunted when the knee is locked (p. 34) and 'screwed home' (p. 53).

94

Ligamentous injuries in flexion

Isolated lesion of the anterior cruciate ligament variation 1 (IL, ACL, Vl)

Isolated lesion of the anterior cruciate ligament variation 1, IL ACL Vl, corresponds to a ligamentous injury in medial rotation (p. 94): injury to the anterior cruciate ligament ACL is isolated, with no lesion in the peripheral structures.

Pathogenesis

The site of involvement (Figure 5.26) covers the anterior half of the intercalary compartment. The trigger mechanism (Figures 5.24 and 5.25) involves no direct contact, but results from twisting of the knee in varus-flexion/medial rotation VrFMR[25] while supporting weight[26].

The typical ACL lesion is obvious or concealed depending on whether or not the synovial membrane is involved. The intrasynovial lesion is localized in the upper or middle part and may be indicated by a haematoma. The obvious lesion with rupture of the synovium produces different signs depending on whether the lesion is high, middle or low. High tears can remain hidden for a long time because they are in a very deep region, difficult to examine: the femoral insertion is located very posterior on the medial facet of lateral femoral condyle (p. 17). The tear in the middle of the ligament, (the most frequent in the adult) results in shredding, and disinsertion on the floor (the lesion of children and adolescents) is occasionally accompanied by avulsion of bone.

When limited to an ACL deficit, abnormal mobility (Figure 5.26) is characterized by normal medial rotation MR and anterior subluxation of the lateral tibial condyle ASL LTC[27].

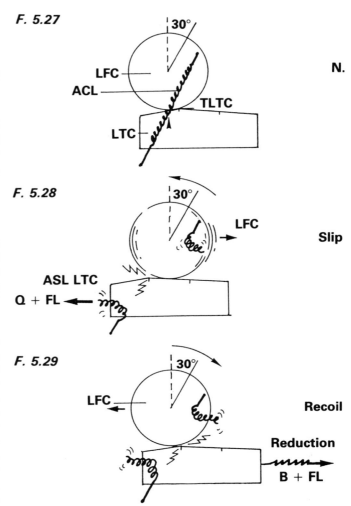

F. 5.27

N.

F. 5.28

Slip

F. 5.29

Recoil

Reduction

By acting as a vascular and protective sheath (pp. 14 and 17), the synovium limits the risk of degeneration. Ceiling tears of the ACL are partially degenerative with the sheath clinging to and being nourished by the posterior cruciate ligament PCL. Middle tears of the ACL are rapidly and totally degenerative, with the ACL being reduced to a bit of ligamentous debris remaining at its insertions. ACL disinsertion from the floor is rarely degenerative, because of the potential consolidation offered by avulsion of bone.

Clinical examination

The interview reveals a history of a 'swollen knee' related to a serious ligamentous injury (p. 63) and possibly haemarthrosis[28] with aspiration having

---

25 Essentially, twisting results from medial rotation with excessive demands resulting in a delay in necessary lateral rotation at the approach to extension (p. 40): the 'fragile' ACL is therefore predisposed to stretching lesions because insufficient unwinding of the two cruciate ligaments does not enable it to recover its stretching potential.

26 The opposing movement occurs when the tibia and foot constitute a single unit fixed to the ground and the femur-pelvis-trunk unit is brought into sudden rotary movement toward the supporting leg. This sprain is illustrated by two examples: the soccer player (Figure 5.24) kicking a cross shot while the supporting foot is held tight to the ground by a cleated shoe; and the skier (Figure 5.25) who twists forward and falls toward the outside of the supporting leg (fronts of skis crossed), with the supporting leg held in place by the tip of the ski planted in the snow.

27 When freed from the anterior cruciate ligament, the lateral femoral condyle LFC can pass over the top of the lateral tibial condyle TLTC at 30° of flexion in medial rotation MR (Figure 3.23).

---

28 Since the haemarthrosis cannot evacuate into soft tissue if there is no peripheral lesion, the increase in volume is usually immediate and extensive in an isolated lesion of the ACL accompanied by rupture of the synovium or avulsion of a fragment of bone.

been carried out (p. 81). Examination findings are astonishingly normal[29], except for the possibility of moderate or extensive pivot shift (PS = ++ to +++, p. 74) with vigorous response (Figures 5.27–5.29 and 4.25).

Special examinations

Opaque arthrography is normal. Arthroscopy (p. 84) confirms the lesion of the ACL.

Course

Decompensation of uninjured peripheral structures is slow, but occurs more rapidly in the individuals subject to the critical constraints of sports or of certain occupations (p. 53 and Note 71).

As a rule: the handicap is zero (H = 0) and remains so for a long time under certain conditions[30]; and the first consultation with a specialist occurs several years after the initial accident (CS = years).

Anterolateral laxity (ALL)

ALL results from a ligamentous injury in medial rotation (p. 94): injury to the anterior cruciate ligament ACL is associated with a lesion to anterolateral peripheral structure.

Pathogenesis
The site of involvement (Figures 5.30 and 5.31) covers the anterior half of the intercalary compartment and the anterior third of the lateral compartment.

The trigger mechanism involves no direct contact, but results from twisting of the knee in varus-flexion/medial rotation VrFMR with support[31].

---

29 The integrity of the peripheral structures; particularly the medial back corner MBC and the lateral front corner LFC makes up for the insufficiency of the ACL (p. 47).

30 A falsely reassuring condition is the rule, as a result of minor increases in musculature and reduction in the physical requirements of the individual's occupation or sport: to the same extent, instability (p. 00) can pass unperceived for a long time, leading to an apparent cure.

31 The opposing movement is similar to that of the isolated lesion of the ACL (p. 95): the preceding examples of the soccer player and skier (Figures 5.24 and 5.25) are included within the general framework of sudden changes of direction toward the side of the supporting foot, with medial rotation always being stronger in anterolateral laxity.

32 The ACL (p. 17) is more or less degenerated depending on the extent of the injury to the synovium (p. 95).

33 The LFC (p. 18 and Note 16) is distended at the deep sheath of its tibial insertion.

34 The LM (p. 16) is torn or disinserted (p. 89), a probable consequence of the trauma connected with dislocation.

35 When freed from the ACL, the medial femoral condyle MFC can roll abnormally on the posterior facet of the tibial condyle at 30° of flexion in medial rotation (Figure 3.23).

The typical combination of lesions (Figures 5.30 and 5.31) affects the anterior cruciate ligament ACL[32], the lateral front corner LFc[33] and the lateral meniscus LM[34].

Abnormal mobility connected with deficiency connected with the lateral (p. 41) and rotary (p. 47) stabilizers has two characteristics:

● Anterior subluxation of the tibial intercondylar space ASL TICS (Figure 5.30).

● A shift of the zero axis of rotation (O) (p. 42 and Figures 3.21 and 3.22) rearward and inward, in other words toward uninjured capsular and ligamentous structures, an increase in medial rotation MHR, a lateral opening—medial rotation LO MR and an anterior subluxation of the lateral tibial condyle ASL LTC[35] (Figure 5.31).

F. 5.30

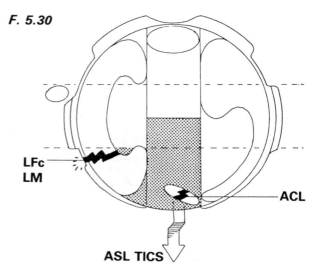

F. 5.31

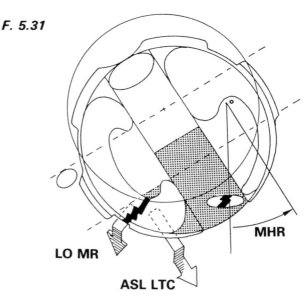

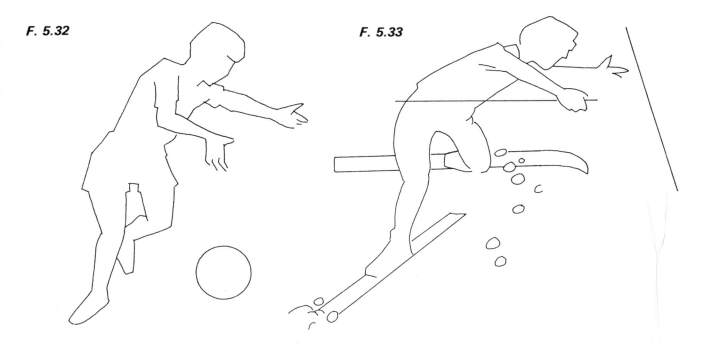

F. 5.32

F. 5.33

Clinical examination

The interview becomes explicit at the indication of the medial rotary dislocation (p. 64), having occurred a number of times following a serious ligamentous injury (p. 93).

Other than the pathognomonic pivot shift test the examination does not produce significant results:

- Varus-medial rotation (p. 72) is weak (VrMR = +).

- Anterior drawer sign—rotation O (p. 72) is weak (ADRO = +).

- Pivot shift (p. 74) is significant (PS = +++) with vigorous response as a result of resistance produced by the medial compartment and the deterioration of the lateral compartment.

Special examinations

Opaque arthrography (p. 81) is used in examination for a disinsertion of the posterior horn of the medial meniscus PHMM[36] which could be reinserted.

Arthroscopy (p. 84) confirms the lesion of the ACL.

---

36 The decoadaptation of the medial compartment as a ricochet effect after dislocation of the lateral compartment, makes disinsertion of the posterior horn of the medial meniscus more likely. PHMM becomes disconnected from its posterior attachments because of the asynchronism that results: the anterior restraint of the medial meniscopatellar ligament MMPL (p. 35) overcomes the posterior recall of the medial dynamic mooring MDM (p. 45).

37 The course can be accelerated by ill-timed surgery with inappropriate surgical acts: meniscectomy without restoration of the ligaments; and a lateral approach to the ileotibial band by horizontal incision (pp. 18 and 19), touching on the part of the superficial sheath of the lateral front corner LFc which is, in principle, spared any damage.

Course

Decompensation of uninjured peripheral structures is slow, but occurs more rapidly than in the isolated lesion of the ACL (p. 95) because it is already initiated by the lesion to the lateral compartment[37].

As a rule, the handicap is slight (H = +) and remains for some time. First consultation with a specialist occurs one year after the initial accident (CS = one year).

Posteromedial laxity version 1 (PML V1)

PML V1 results from a ligamentous injury in medial rotation (p. 93), but with an entity that is subject to discussion because it is not precisely determined and it is paradoxical in appearance: in fact, the lesion of the posteromedial peripheral structures (Figure 3.34) produces a 'false' anterior drawer sign—medial rotation ADMR that occurs as the price of reducing a posterior subluxation of the medial tibial condyle.

Anteromedial laxity (AML)

AML results from a ligamentous injury in lateral rotation (p. 93): injury to the anterior cruciate ligament ACL is associated with a lesion in the posteromedial peripheral structures.

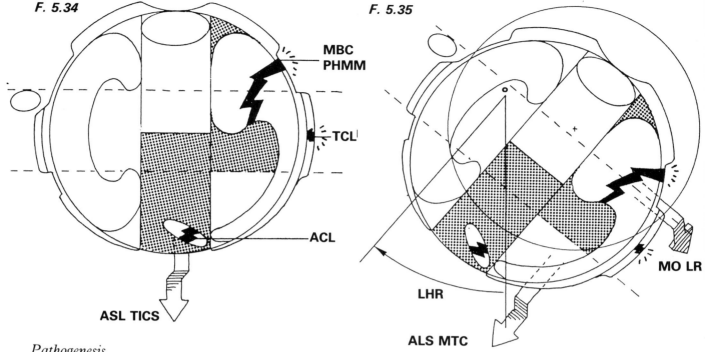

F. 5.34

MBC
PHMM

TCL

ACL

ASL TICS

F. 5.35

LHR

MO LR

ALS MTC

Pathogenesis

The site of involvement (Figures 5.34 and 5.35) covers the anterior half of the intercalary compartment, the middle third and posterior third of the medial compartment. The trigger mechanism (Figures 5.32 and 5.33) usually involves no direct contact[38] but results from twisting of the knee in valgus-flexion-lateral rotation VlFLR[39] with support[40]. The typical combination of lesions (Figures 5.34 and 5.35) involves the anterior cruciate ligament ACL[41], the medial back corner MBC[42], the medial meniscus MM[43] and the tibial collateral ligament TCL[44].

Abnormal mobility linked to deficiency of the lateral (p. 43) and rotary (p. 46) stabilizers is characterized by:

● Anterior subluxation of the tibial intercondylar space ASL TICS (Figure 5.34).

● A shift of the zero axis of rotation O (p. 42 and Figures 3.21 and 3.22) rearward and outward (in other words toward uninjured capsular and ligamentous structures), a lateral hyper-rotation LHR, a medial opening-lateral rotation MO LR and anterior subluxation of the medial tibial condyle ASL MTC (Figure 5.35). Normal medial rotation MR and anterior subluxation of the lateral tibial condyle ASL LTC (Figure 5.26).

Clinical examination

The interview is explicit by its description of lateral rotary instability (p. 64), with an 'uninterrupted' chronic continuation of a serious ligamentous injury (p. 93).

Examination results are demonstrative:

● Lateral hyper-rotation (p. 70) is weak or moderate (LHR = + to ++).

● Valgus-lateral rotation (p. 71) is weak or moderate (VlLR = + to ++).

---

38 The direct contact mechanism implies direct or distant violence: the impact occurs on the posterolateral surface of the knee or on the medial border of the arch or ball of the foot.

39 The twisting of the knee results from both the valgus and lateral rotation whose excessive demands upon approaching extension anticipate its own stretching possibilities to the point of locking (p. 34): the ACL is particularly predisposed to a stretching lesion on the medial facet of the lateral femoral condyle, which serves as a sawhorse.

40 The twisting occurs when the tibia and foot constitute a single unit fixed to the ground and the femur-pelvis-trunk unit is brought into sudden rotary movement directed toward the side opposite the supporting leg. This sprain is illustrated by two examples: the soccer player (Figure 5.32) faking out an opponent by shifting to the inside, in other words moving away from the supporting foot while that foot is held tight to the ground by a cleated shoe; the skier (Figure 5.33) who twists forward and toward the inside of the supporting leg (backs of skis cross), which is held in place by the support ski.

41 The ACL (p. 17) is totally degenerated as the sequela of a tear that most often occurs in the middle of a ligament (p. 94).

42 The MBC (p. 20) is extremely distended in its anterior part, forming a dehiscent and prominent pouch when examined with a haemostat introduced by anterior arthrotomy up to the posterior limit of the tibial collateral ligament.

43 The MM (p. 17) is torn as well as disinserted, but with the posterior horn PHMM (Figure 5.3) always affected.

44 The TCL (p. 20) is slightly distended from a juxtameniscal tear or a femoral disinsertion.

- The anterior drawer sign—rotation O (p. 72) is weak or moderate (ADRO = + to ++), increasing in anterior drawer sign—lateral rotation (ADLR = ++) and being eliminated in anterior drawer sign—medial rotation (ADMR = O).

- The pivot shift (p. 74) is weak (PS = +) with slack response connected with release of the medial compartment.

Additional radiological examination
The anterior drawer sign—rotation O test (p. 72) (ADRO) is carried out and used to measure the radiodynamic drawer sign RxD obtained.

Special examinations
Opaque arthrography (p. 81) makes it possible to differentiate between a tear and a disinsertion, in order to provide an indication of possible reinsertion of the posterior horn of the medial meniscus PHMM. Arthroscopy (p. 84) is of no use.

Course
There is rapid decompensation of uninjured peripheral structures. As a rule, there is a heavy handicap (H = +++), to the point of ruling out any resumption of sports and occasionally of work. The first consultation with a specialist occurs several weeks after the initial accident (CS = weeks).

Posterolateral laxity version 1 (PLL Vl)

PLL Vl is first indicated by difficulties in diagnosis and treatment. It results from a ligamentous injury in lateral rotation (p. 93): injury to the posterolateral peripheral structures contrasts with the apparent lack of injury to the posterior cruciate ligament PCL.

Pathogenesis
The site of involvement (Figure 5.36) covers the posterior third of the lateral compartment. The trigger mechanism involves no direct contact, but results from twisting of the knee in valgus-flexion/lateral rotation VlFLR with support[45].

The typical combination of lesions (Figure 5.31) includes the lateral back corner LBC[46], lateral

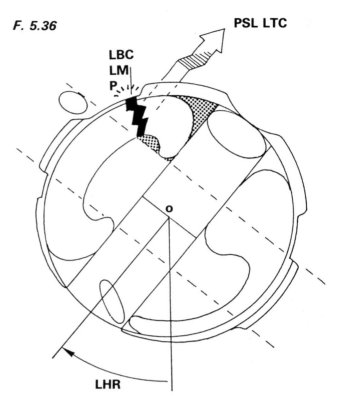

F. 5.36

meniscus LM[47] and popliteal P[48]. Abnormal mobility (Figure 5.36) is connected with deficiency in the lateral (p. 41) and rotary (p. 47) stabilizers and is aggravated by failure of the popliteal (p. 59 and Note 93). The outstanding feature is an imperceptible shift of the axis of rotation (p. 42 and Notes 33 and 34), lateral hyper-rotation LHR and a posterior subluxation of the lateral tibial condyle PSL LTC.

Clinical examination
The interview is summarized by lateral rotary instability and posterolateral pain which has persisted from the time of a serious ligamentous injury (p. 93).

Examination results are poor and difficult to interpret:

- Lateral hyper-rotation (p. 70) weak or moderate (LHR = + to ++) is taken into account if all anteromedial laxity tests are negative (p. 97).

- The Big Toe Test BT (p. 71) sometimes supplies the only significant indications.

---

45 The trigger mechanism is the same as that for anteromedial laxity: the preceding examples of the soccer player and skier (Figures 5.32 and 5.33) fall in the same category of sudden changes of direction toward the side opposite the supporting foot, and always include more extreme lateral rotation in posterolateral laxity.

46 The LBC (p. 17) is extremely distended, a sequela to a tear in the fibular collateral ligament (short) FCL-S.

47 The LM (p. 20) is torn as well as disinserted, but always accompanied by involvement of the posterior horn PHLM (p. 89).

48 The P (p. 30) is elongated, a sequela to a rupture of the tendinomuscular unit because of rearward movement of the lateral tibial condyle.

- The posterior drawer sign—rotation O (p. 72) is zero (PDRO = O), and appears weak in posterior drawer sign—lateral rotation (PDLR = +) and is zero in posterior drawer sign—medial rotation (PDMR = O).

- Reverse pivot shift (p. 74) is more or less evident (RPS = + to ++ to +++) with a more or less vigorous response.

Special examinations
Arthroscopy (p. 84) makes it possible to distinguish between disinsertion and tear of the posterior horn of the lateral meniscus PHLM in order to indicate the possibilities of reinsertion. Arthroscopy is of no use.

Course
There is fairly rapid decompensation of uninjured peripheral structures. As a rule, the handicap is medium (H = ++) to the point of only becoming evident during sports; and the first consultation with a specialist occurs in the months following the initial accident (CS = months).

Isolated lesion of the posterior cruciate ligament (IL PCL)

Isolated lesion of the posterior cruciate ligament results from a ligamentous injury in neutral rotation (p. 94); injury to the posterior cruciate ligament PCL is isolated with no lesions in the peripheral structures.

Pathogenesis
The site of involvement (Figure 5.38) covers the posterior half of the intercalary compartment.

The trigger mechanism (Figure 5.37) involves direct contact, resulting from the knee being forced backward when in 90° flexion with the heel blocked: the direct violence is anterior, with the point of impact located at the level of the anterior tibial tuberosity[49].

The typical lesion (Figure 5.38) is, in principle, evident because of the tear on the ceiling or in the middle of the ligament, or disinsertion on the floor occasionally accompanied by avulsion of bone[50].

---

[49] This type of forced movement happens to the automobile driver (Figure 5.37) or the motorcyclist whose flexed knee in neutral rotation hits the dashboard or safety bar: the anteroposterior direction results in the proximal end of the tibia being forced rearward.

[50] In practice, it is difficult to specify whether the injury is high, medium or low, no matter what observation procedure is used. This makes it difficult to choose the surgical approach and therapeutic procedure.

Abnormal mobility (Figure 5.38), linked to simple deficiency of the PCL, is characterized by posterior subluxation of the tibial intercondylar space PSL TICS. The vascularization possibilities of PCL (p. 17 and Note 15) and the consolidation possibilities provided by avulsion of bone, limit the risk of degeneration.

Clinical examination
The interview establishes the link between a pain in the popliteal fossa and a serious ligamentous injury (p. 93), more or less overlooked in the tumult of the initial accident.

F. 5.37

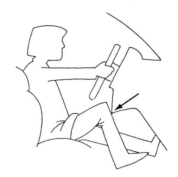

F. 5.38

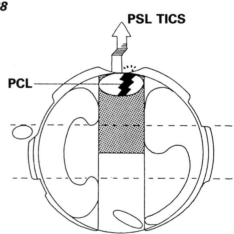

The examination is made evident by the voluntary posterior drawer VPD (p. 69) with disappearance of the anterior tibial tuberosity, and by the posterior drawer sign (p. 72), which is weak or moderate in zero rotation (PDRO = + to ++).

Radiological examination
The posterior drawer sign—rotation O PDRO (p. 81) is used to determine the radiodynamic drawer sign RxD.

Special examinations
Opaque arthrography (p. 81) is normal. Arthroscopy (p. 84) confirms the PCL lesion.

Course

There is a very slow decompensation of uninjured peripheral structures, impossible to detect clinically. As a rule, the handicap is negligible (H = ± O) and remains so for a long time under certain conditions[51]. The first consultation with a specialist occurs one or more years after the initial accident (CS = one or more years).

Ligamentous Injury in Extension

Isolated lesion of the anterior cruciate version 2 (IL ACL V2)

Isolated lesion of the anterior cruciate version 2 results from a ligamentous injury in extension (p. 93): injury to the anterior cruciate ligament ACL is isolated, with no lesion in the peripheral structures.

Variation 2 is identical to variation 1 (p. 95) with the exception of several pathogenetic features: the trigger mechanism (Figure 5.39) involves no direct contact, but results from forced movement of the knee in extension[52] with support[53].

Posterior laxity (PL)

PL results from a ligamentous injury in extension (p. 93); injury to the posterior cruciate ligament PCL is associated with a lesion to the posterior capsule.

Pathogenesis

The site of involvement (Figure 5.41) covers the posterior half of the intercalary compartment and extends into the posterior thirds of the lateral and medial compartments.

The trigger mechanism (Figure 5.40) most often involves direct contact, resulting from forced movement of the knee in extension with the heel

---

51 In fact, the future is mortgaged by the risk of an intercurrent accident, which is an *a priori* danger to the athlete.

52 The forced movement is a result of a sudden body movement beyond normal blocking conditions: the 'fragile' ACL (p. 17) is called into play when it is already at its maximum length (p. 54). These are predisposing conditions for a stretching lesion.

53 The forced movement is produced in suspension, such as the soccer player missing the ball 'on the fly' with a particularly violent attempt to kick it with his instep.

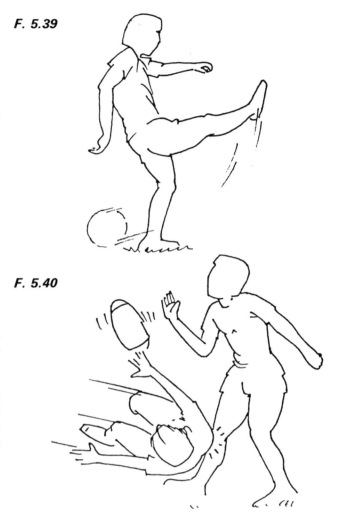

F. 5.39

F. 5.40

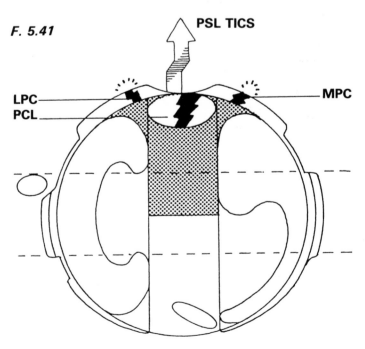

F. 5.41

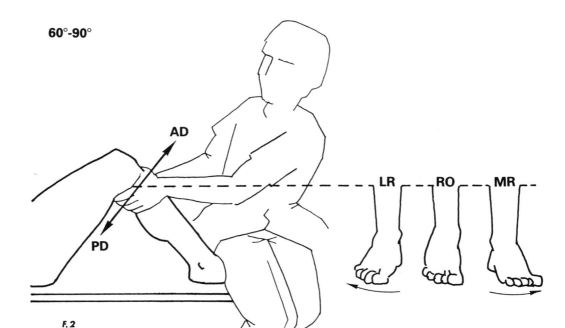

F. 5.42   **60°-90°**

AD
PD
LR   RO   MR
F. 2

blocked[54]: direct violence is anterior with the point of impact on the anterior tibial tuberosity[55].

The typical combination of lesions (Figure 5.41) involves the PCL[56] and the lateral posterior capsule LPC and medial posterior capsule MPC[57]. Normal mobility is characterized by posterior subluxation of the tibial intercondylar space PSL TICS.

Clinical examination
The interview is descriptive by discomfort in the standing at rest position, this position having become painful and unstable following a serious ligamentous injury (p. 93).

The examination is demonstrative:

● Unilateral deformation in genu recurvatum GRv (p. 64) is evident.

● Voluntary posterior drawer VPD (p. 69) with disappearance of the projection of the anterior tibial tuberosity.

● Hyperextension HE (p. 70) is moderate or important (HE = ++ to +++).

● Posterior drawer sign—rotation O PDRO (p. 72) is moderate or important (PDRO = ++ to +++), is recovered in posterior drawer sign—lateral rotation PDLR (PDLR = ++ to +++), and decreases in posterior drawer sign—medial rotation PDMR (PDMR = +) (Figure 5.42).

Additional radiological examination
The posterior drawer sign—rotation O PDRO is reproduced to measure the radiodynamic drawer sign RxD.

Special examinations
Opaque arthrography (p. 81) is normal, with the exception of a possible escape of opaque fluid below the lower limit of the posterior capsule. Arthroscopy (p. 84) confirms the PCL lesion.

Course
There is rapid decompensation of uninjured peripheral structures. As a rule, the handicap is heavy (H = +++), and is incompatible with the resumption of sports and work, and the first consultation with a specialist occurs several weeks after the initial accident (CS = weeks).

---

54 Forced movement beyond normal knee locking (p. 34) to some extent breaks the 'safety lock' which is made up of the PCL and the posterior capsule.

55 Forced movement by anterior contact is fairly frequent in sports: the rugby player (Figure 5.40), heeling out on a pass, with the leg passively extended at the hip and receiving the sudden block or fall of an opponent.

56 The PCL (p. 17) is partially degenerated, most often as a result of disinsertion on the floor (p. 100).

57 The LPC and MPC are distended as the sequela to femoral or tibial disinsertion, or a tear in the middle.

Posterolateral laxity version 2 (PLL V2)

Posterolateral laxity version 2 is first indicated by rapid deterioration. It results from a ligamentous injury in extension (p. 94): injury to the posterior cruciate ligament PCL is associated with a lesion in the posterolateral peripheral structures.

Pathogenesis

The site of involvement (Figures 5.44 and 5.45) covers the posterior half of the intercalary compartment, and the middle and posterior thirds of the lateral compartment.

The trigger mechanism (Figure 5.43) involves direct contact and results from forced movement of the knee in extension with support[58]: the direct violence is lateral with an anteromedial point of impact[59].

Typical combinations of lesions (Figures 5.44 and 5.45) involve the posterior cruciate ligament PCL and the lateral posterior capsule LPC[60], the lateral back corner LBC and the lateral meniscus LM[61], the popliteal muscle P[62], and the fibular collateral ligament (long) FCL-L[63].

The abnormal mobility linked to deficiency in the lateral (p. 41) and rotary (p. 47) stabilizers is characterized by:

● Lateral opening LO and posterior subluxation of the tibial intercondylar space PSL TICS (Figure 5.44).

● An imperceptible shift in the axis of rotation (p. 42 and Notes 33 and 34), lateral hyper-rotation LHR, lateral opening—lateral rotation LO LR and posterior subluxation of the lateral tibial condyle PSL LTC (Figure 5.45).

Clinical examination

The interview is explicit through the obvious connection between a serious ligamentous injury (p. 93) combined with dislocation and posterolateral pain.

---

58 Forced movement results from pure varus pushed beyond normal knee locking (p. 34), consequently breaking the various elements that participate in posterolateral capsular and ligamentous resistance.

59 Forced movement from anteromedial contact is possible in sports: for example the centre forward (Figure 5.43) whose support leg is hit by a diving goalie.

60 The injured condition of the PCL and the LPC are identical to those described in posterior laxity (p. 102).

61 The conditions of the LBC and the LM are identical to those described in PLL V1 (p. 99 and Notes 46 and 47).

62 The P (p. 30) is elongated, as a result of a femoral disinsertion or rupture in the middle.

63 The FCL-L (p. 18) is distended, resulting from a juxtameniscal tear or a femoral or fibular disinsertion.

F. 5.43

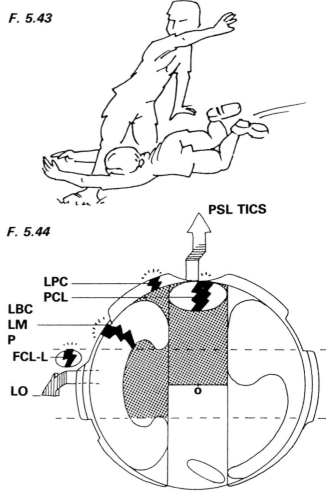

F. 5.44

PSL TICS

LPC
PCL
LBC
LM
P
FCL-L
LO

F. 5.45

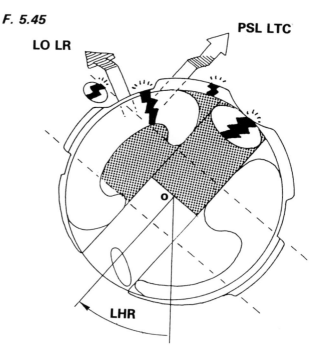

PSL LTC
LO LR
LHR

The examination is demonstrative:

- Unilateral deformation in genu varus GVr and genu recurvatum GRv (p. 64) is visible when standing on both feet and is aggravated by walking.

- Voluntary posterior drawer VPD (p. 69) obliterates the projection of the anterior tibial tuberosity.

- Hyperextension HE (p. 70) is weak or moderate (HE = + to ++).

- Lateral hyper-rotation LHR (p. 70) is weak or moderate (LHR = + to ++).

- Varus-extension VrE (p. 72) is weak or moderate (VrE = + to ++).

- The Big Toe Test BT (p. 71) reproduces deformation and dislocation conditions.

- Varus-lateral rotation VrLR (p. 72) is moderate or important (VrLR = ++ to +++).

- Posterior drawer sign—rotation O PDRO (p. 72) is moderate, accented in posterior drawer sign—lateral rotation (PDLR = +++), and reduced in posterior drawer sign—medial rotation (PDMR = +).

Additional radiological examination
Posterior drawer sign—rotation O PDRO (p. 72) is used to measure the radiodynamic drawer sign RxD.

Special examinations
Opaque arthrography (p. 81) may differentiate between disinsertion and tearing of the posterior horn of the lateral meniscus PHLM, which can be disinserted. Arthroscopy (p. 84) is of no value.

Course
There is rapid decompensation in genu varus GVr[64], always maintaining the advantage of protecting healthy medial peripheral structures.

As a rule the handicap is heavy (H = +++), and is incompatible with resumption of sports and work; and the first consultation with a specialist occurs in the weeks following the initial accident (CS = weeks).

Anteroposterolateral laxity (APLL)

Anteroposterolateral laxity results from a ligamentous injury in extension (p. 101): injury to the central pivot is associated with a lesion in the lateral peripheral structure.

Pathogenesis
The site of involvement (Figures 5.47–5.49) covers the whole intercalary compartment and the lateral compartment.

The trigger mechanism (Figure 5.46) involves direct contact and results from forced movement of the knee in extension with support[65]: direct violence is lateral with a medial point of impact[66].

The typical combination of lesions (Figures 5.47–5.49) is extensive, involving the anterior cruciate ligament ACL, the lateral front corner LFc and the lateral meniscus LM[67], the posterior cruciate ligament PCL, the lateral posterior capsule LPC, the lateral back corner LBC, the lateral meniscus LM, the popliteal P and the fibular collateral ligament (long) FCL-L[68]; the biceps B[69] and occasionally the common peroneal nerve CPN[70], the iliotibial aponeurosis ITA[71].

Abnormal mobility is characterized by:

- Lateral opening LO in extension, anterior subluxation of the tibial intercondylar space ASL TICS and posterior subluxation of the tibial intercondylar space PSL TICS (Figure 5.47).

A shift in the axis of rotation O (p. 42 and Notes 33 and 34) within the medial compartment (in other words toward the uninjured capsular and ligamentous structures); medial hyper-rotation MHR, lateral opening—medial rotation LO MR, and anterior subluxation of the lateral tibial condyle ASL LTC; lateral hyper-rotation LHR, lateral opening—lateral rotation LO LR and posterior subluxation of the lateral tibial condyle PSL LTC (Figures 5.48 and 5.49).

---

64 The failure of lateral peripheral structures, including the fibular collateral ligament FCL-L, frees varus demands which depend on weight-bearing (p. 60).

65 Forced movement results from pure varus pushed beyond the conditions of normal knee locking (p. 34): the FCL-L and the LBC back up the PCL in a demand for optimal stretching, creating conditions for a stretching lesion before ACL and the other elements yield under the same conditions.

66 Forced movement resulting from medial contact is typical of traffic accidents and possibly sports such as cross-country motorcycle racing (Figure 5.46): the motorcycle falls against the leg which is providing support.

67 The conditions of ACL, LFc and LM injuries is identical to that described for anterolateral laxity (p. 96).

68 The conditions of injury for the whole group consisting of the PCL, LPC, LBC, LM, P and FCL-L is identical to that described for posterolateral laxity version 2 (p. 103).

69 The B (pp. 28 and 29) is elongated, the sequela to a rupture at the tendinomuscular junction or in the middle.

70 The CPN is elongated or ruptured, with the latter being most frequent, and disguised because its focal point is some distance from the knee and paralysis occurs which is often impossible to reverse.

71 The ITA (p. 18), a constituent part of the fascia lata (p. 27), is distended or intact.

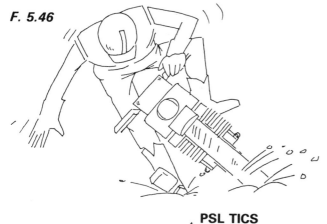

Clinical examination

The interview establishes the connection between limping and a serious ligamentous injury (p. 93).

The examination is demonstrative:

Unilateral deformation in genu varus GVr and genu recurvatum GRv (p. 64) are visible when the patient is standing on both feet and is aggravated by walking. There is indication of an opening of the posterolateral interline. There is voluntary posterior drawer VPD (p. 69) with disappearance of the anterior tibial tuberosity, resulting in confusion with the voluntary anterior drawer VAD (p. 69) which renders it more prominent.

- Hyperextension HE (p. 70) is moderate (HE = ++) and is indicated by posterolateral opening.

- Lateral hyper-rotation LHR (p. 70) is important (LHR = +++) in relation to the increase in medial rotation, which is difficult to evaluate—varus-extension VrE (p. 72) is moderate or important (VrE = ++ to +++). The drawer sign—extension DE (p. 72) is manifest.

- The Big Toe Test BT (p. 71) reproduces the conditions of deformation and limping.

- Varus—lateral rotation VrLR (p. 72) is moderate or important (VrLR = ++ to +++) whereas it is no more than moderate in varus—medial rotation VrMR (p. 72) (VrMR = ++).

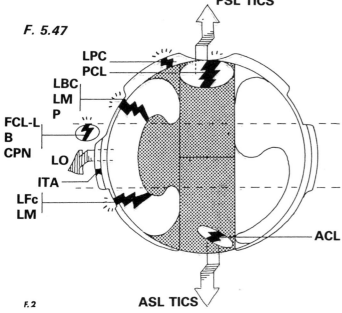

F. 5.47

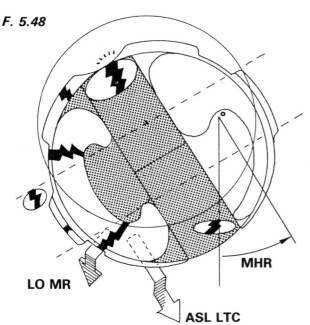

F. 5.48

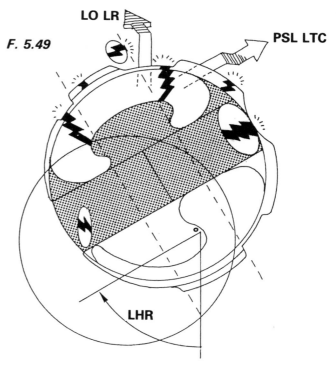

F. 5.49

- The anterior drawer sign—rotation O ADRO (p. 72) is moderate (ADRO = ++), diminished in anterior drawer sign—lateral rotation (ADLR = +), and is found in anterior drawer sign—medial rotation (ADMR = ++). The posterior drawer sign — rotation O PDRO (p. 72) is moderate (PDRO = ++), accentuated in posterior drawer sign—lateral rotation (PDLR = +++), and diminished in posterior drawer sign—medial rotation (PDMR = +).

- Pivot shift (p. 74) is difficult to distinguish from reverse pivot shift (p. 75) with what is, in principle, a vigorous response (PS RPS).

Additional radiological examination

It shows (p. 80) lateral interline opening LIO and reveals (p. 81) the radiodynamic opening RxO and the double radiodynamic drawer sign RxD.

Special examinations

Special examinations are superfluous.

Course

There is very rapid decompensation in genu varus GVr[72], always maintaining the advantage of protecting uninjured medial peripheral structures.

As a rule the handicap is very heavy (H = ++++) to the point of hindering daily existence, and the first consultation with a specialist is close to ten days after the initial accident (CS about the 10th day).

Posteromedial laxity version 2 (PML V2)

Primary posteromedial laxity version 2 is a rare disorder. It results from a ligamentous injury in extension (p. 101): it is probably a sort of modification with some of the elements of anteroposteromedial laxity.

Anteroposteromedial laxity (APML)

Anteroposteromedial laxity results from a ligamentous injury in extension (p. 101): injury to the central pivot is associated with a lesion in the medial peripheral structures.

Pathogenesis

The site of involvement (Figures 5.52–5.54) covers the whole intercalary compartment and the medial compartment.

The trigger mechanism (Figures 5.50 and 5.51) involves no direct contact, but results from forced movement from the knee in extension with support[73]: direct violence is lateral with a lateral point of impact[74].

The typical combination of lesions (Figures 5.52–5.54) is extensive: the anterior cruciate ligament ACL, the medial back corner MBC, the medial meniscus MM and the tibial collateral ligament TCL[75]; the posterior cruciate ligament PCL and the medial posterior capsule MPC[76], the semimembranous muscle SM[77].

Abnormal mobility is characterized by:

- Medial opening MO in extension, anterior subluxation of the tibial intercondylar space ASL TICS and posterior subluxation of the tibial intercondylar space PSL TICS (Figure 5.52).

- A shift in the axis of rotation O (p. 42 and Notes 33 and 34) in the lateral compartment, in other words toward the uninjured capsular and ligamentous structures; a medial hyper-rotation MHR, medial opening—medial rotation MO MR, and posterior subluxation of the medial tibial condyle PSL MTC; lateral hyper-rotation LHR, medial opening—lateral rotation MO LR, and anterior subluxation of the medial tibial condyle ASL MTC (Figures 5.53 and 5.54).

Clinical examination

The interview is summarized by instability following a serious ligamentous injury (p. 93).

The examination is demonstrative:

- Unilateral deformation in genu recurvatum GRv (p. 64) is evident. There is voluntary posterior

---

73 The forced movement results in pure valgus pushed beyond normal knee locking (p. 34): the LLI and the MBC back up the PCL in a demand for maximum stretching, creating conditions for a stretching injury before the ACL and other elements yield under these same conditions.

74 Forced movement resulting from lateral contact is frequent in practice as well as in warm-up and normal participation, as is illustrated by two examples: hitting another player's leg instead of the ball when parrying in soccer (Figure 5.50); and judo throws (Figure 5.51) that involve 'blocking' to put the opponent off balance.

75 The conditions of injury to the whole group of ACL, MBC, MM and TCL is identical to that described in anteromedial laxity (p. 97).

76 The conditions of PCL and MBC injury are identical to that described in posterior laxity (p. 101).

77 The SM (p. 30) is elongated, a consequence of disinsertion or a rupture of the insertion complex.

---

72 The failing of lateral peripheral structures including the fibular collateral ligament (long) FCL-L, and particularly the fascia lata FL through the iliotibial aponeurosis ITA, frees varus demands that are dependent on weight-bearing (p. 61).

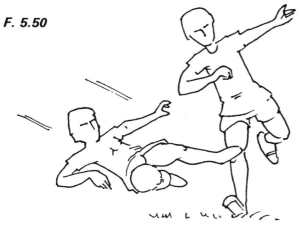

F. 5.50

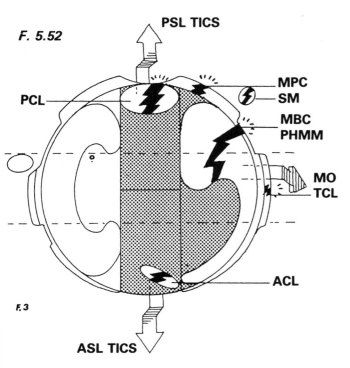

F. 5.51

drawer VPD (p. 69) with disappearance of the anterior tibial tuberosity, resulting in confusion with the voluntary anterior drawer VAD (p. 69) which renders it more prominent.

● Hyperextension HE (p. 70) is moderate (HE = ++). Lateral hyper-rotation (p. 70) is moderate (LHR = ++) in relation to an increase in medial rotation that is difficult to evaluate.

F. 5.53

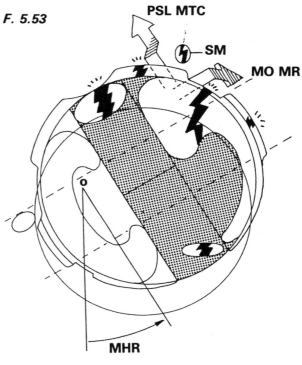

F. 5.52

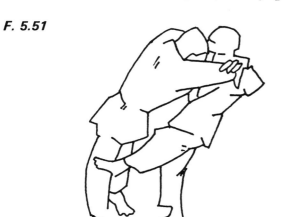

F. 5.54

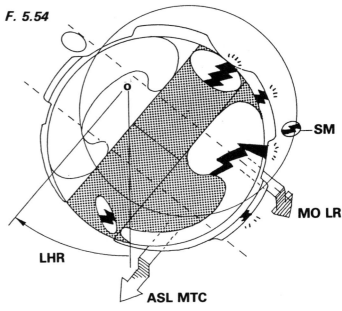

- Valgus extension (p. 71) is moderate or important (VlE = ++ to +++). The lateral drawer sign DE (p. 71) is manifest.

- Valgus—lateral rotation and valgus—medial rotation (p. 72) are moderate or important (VlLR and VlMR = ++ to +++).

- The anterior drawer sign—rotation O (p. 72) is moderate (ADRO = ++), accentuated in anterior drawer sign—lateral rotation (ADLR = +++), and diminished or recovered in anterior drawer sign—medial rotation (ADMR = + to ++). The posterior drawer sign—rotation O (p. 72) is moderate (PDRO = ++), decreased in posterior drawer sign—lateral rotation (PDLR = +), and accentuated in posterior drawer sign—medial rotation (PDMR = +++).

- Pivot shift (p. 74) is weak (PS = +) with a very weak response.

Additional radiological examination
Radiological examination (p. 81) shows radiodynamic opening RxO and double radiodynamic drawer sign RxD.

Specialized examination
Specialized examinations are superfluous.

Course
Decompensation in genu varus GVr is retarded as long as the integrity of the lateral peripheral structures can contain varus demands (p. 60).

As a rule the handicap is paradoxically light (H = +) and remains so for some time. The first consultation with a specialist occurs one year after the initial accident (CS = one year).

CHRONIC LESIONS:

	Trigger mechanism	Type of injury						Abnormal mobility		Interview
IL ACL VI p.95	Flexion Medial Rotation Support	ACL							ASL LTC	Swollen Knee (Haemarthrosis)
ALL p.96	Flexion Medial Rotation Support	ACL	LFC	LM			MHR	LORI	ASL LTC ASL TICS	Rotary Dislocation
AML p.97	Flexion Lateral Rotation Support	ACL	MBC	MM		TCL	LHR	MORE	ASL MTC ASL TICS ASL LTC	Rotary Instability
PLL VI p.99	Flexion Lateral Rotation Support		LBC	LM	P		LHR		PSL LTC	Rotary Instability
IL PCL p.100	Flexion 90° Rotation O Countersupport Anterior Contact	PCL							PSL TICS	Posterior Pain
IL ACL V2 p.101	Extension Suspension	ACL							ASL LTC	Swollen Knee (Haemarthrosis)
PL p.101	Extension Countersupport Anterior Contact	PCL LPC MPC							PSL TICS	Posterior Instability Posterior Pain
PLL V2 p.103	Extension Support Anteromedial Contact	PCL LPC	LBC	LM	P	FCL-L	LHR	LO LORE	PSL TICS PSL TICS	Post.Dislocation Posterolateral Pain
APLL p.104	Extension Support Lateromedial Contact	ACL PCL LPC	LFC LBC	LM LM	P	FCL-L B CPN ITA	MHR LHR	LORI LO LORE	ASL LTC ASL TICS PSL TICS PSL LTC	Limping
APML p.106	Extension Support Lateroposterior Contact	ACL PCL MPC	MBC	MM		TCL SM	LHR MHR	MORE MO MORI	ASL MTC ASL TICS PSL TICS	Instability

109

SUMMARY CLASSIFICATION

Examination				Arthrography	Arthroscopy	Handicap(H)	First consultation specialist(CS)
'NORMAL' PS = ++ to +++				N	yes	0	Years
VrMR = + ADRO = + PS = +++				PHMM	yes	+	1 year
LHR = + to ++ V1LR = + to ++ ADRO = + to ++ PS = +	ADLR = ++	ADMR = O	RxD	PHMM	no	+++	Weeks
LHR = + to ++ BT PDRO = O RPS = +, ++ to +++	PDLR = +	PDMR = O		PHLM	no	++	Months
VPD PDRO = + to ++			RxD	N	yes	±	1 to several years
'NORMAL' PS = ++ to +++				N	yes	0	Years
GRv VPD HE = ++ to +++ PDRO = ++ to +++	PDLR = ++ to +++	PDMR = +	RxD	N	yes	+++	Weeks
GVr GRv VPD HE = + to ++ LHR = + to ++ VrE = + to ++ BT VrLR = ++ to +++ PDRO = ++	PDLR = +++	PDMR = +	RxD	PHLM	no	+++	Weeks
GVr GRv VPD VAD HE = ++ LHR = +++ VrE = ++ to +++ DE BT VrLR = ++ to +++ ADRO = ++ PDRO = ++ PS RPS	VrMR = ++ to +++ ADLR = + PDLR = +++	ADMR = ++ PDMR =+	LIO RxO RxD RxD	no	no	++++	within 10 days
GRv VPD VAD HE = ++ LHR = ++ V1E = ++ to +++ ADRO = ++ PS = +	ADLR = +++	ADMR = to ++	RxO RxD	no	no	+	1 year

Natural history of chronic lesions

Chronic lesions involve the failure of an inseparable and unified set of functional elements (pp. 50–60). They arise from predisposing mechanical factors or trigger mechanisms, and are usually of three general types. The 'fatigue conditions' linked to abnormal mobility while constraints of the occupation, particularly sports, become excessive (p. 53 and Note 71); the occurrence of an intercurrent ligamentous injury, which is always predisposing even in a benign form; therapeutic errors such as a simple meniscectomy in an isolated lesion of the anterior cruciate, etc.

Once this deterioration begins, the pathological picture will be filled in on the basis of the potential development of the basic injuries (p. 93). These lesions can be listed under two headings:

(1) Lesions undergoing no further development, because the initial injury limits the maximum degree of seriousness:

- Isolated lesion of the posterior cruciate ligament IL PCL (p. 100).
- Anteroposterolateral laxity APLL (p. 104).
- Anteroposteromedial laxity APML (p. 106).

(2) Lesions undergoing further development or combining to form new problems around the posterior cruciate ligament PCL, in other words, around the only elements of the central pivot that maintains, or nearly maintains its integrity (Figure 5.55). These include

- Isolated lesion of the anterior cruciate IL ACL (pp. 95 and 101), as a hinge injury between anterolateral laxity ALL and anteromedial laxity AML, later developing into one or the other.
- Anterolateral laxity ALL (p. 96) combines with the posterolateral PLL (p. 99) to produce the global lateral laxity GLL.
- Anteromedial laxity AML (p. 97) combines with anterolateral laxity ALL (p. 96) to produce the global anterior laxity GAL which is straightforward to diagnose. Signs include mutual development of instability and dislocation, development of significant anterior drawer sign—medial rotation (ADMR = + to ++), along with an increase in pivot shift (PS = ++ to +++), accompanied by loss of vigour.

- Anteromedial laxity AML (p. 97) combines with posterolateral laxity PLL (p. 99), corresponding to the same ligamentous injury as occurs in lateral rotation, and with global crossed laxity GCL that is often difficult to diagnose. In fact if posterolateral pain is a prominent feature, the posterolateral component may escape diagnosis in a summary examination, and may simulate global anterior laxity GAL through a false anterior drawer sign—medial rotation[78].

F. 5.55

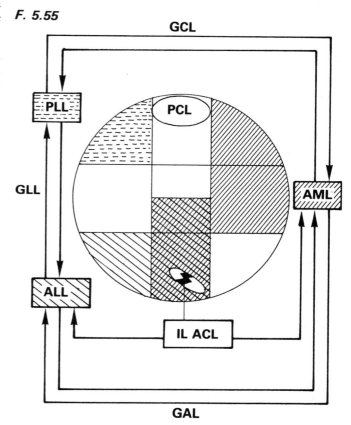

Complications

Patellar imbalance

This is a complication that occurs with ligamentous injury in lateral rotation: anteromedial laxity (p. 98), particularly in its global form, corresponds to one of the dynamic causes of lateral 'malposition' of

---

78 The false ADMR resulting from hypermobility of the lateral area has a number of causes: lateral hyper-rotation as a result of simultaneous posterolateral laxity and anteromedial laxity, the loosening of posterolateral structures (p. 98), particularly with disinsertion of the posterior horn of the lateral meniscus (p. 49) and elongation of the popliteal tendon (p. 59 and Note 93).

the anterior tibial tuberosity ATT that is responsible for frontal patellar imbalance (p. 118 et seq). It occurs whether the patellofemoral joint is initially normal or already predisposed to patellar imbalance.

Abnormal mobility indicates lateral subluxation or lateral dislocation of the patella. Lesions are always chronic and sometimes acute (pp. 118–119), but never pathognomonic of anteromedial laxity.

Since lateral patellar instability simultaneously involves the patellofemoral and tibiofemoral joints it is difficult to diagnose, and there is a risk of missing:

● The seriousness of the dislocation (p. 122 and Note 1) which may be mistaken for laxity;

● The bayonet sign (Figure 5.56) which enables us to recognize the lateral 'malposition' of the anterior tibial tuberosity (pp. 66–68), probably masked by the predominance of laxity, while x-rays of patellar imbalance (p. 81) remain indeterminant.

Tibiofemoral bone and cartilage lesions

Medial compartment
This is a fairly frequent and stereotyped complication of a ligamentous injury in lateral rotation: anteromedial laxity (p. 98) is particularly involved in its global form (p. 111), with the possibility that the bone and cartilage lesion could always be recent, in other words realized in fresh condition (p. 93).

Abnormal mobility with anterior subluxation of the medial tibial condyle ASL MTC (Figure 5.57) takes on major importance with dilaceration of the posterior horn of the medial meniscus PHMM[79] accompanying a tearing loose of the posterior capsule-periosteum[80].

The osteocartilaginous lesions are pathognomonic. Femoral lesions (Figure 5.58) are focused on the posterior half of the medial femoral condyle MFC, but also characteristically along the border with the intercondylar notch ICN: the initial appearance can be summarized as the superimposition of small transverse streaks[81], while ulceration occurs further forward as a result of an actual explosion of cartilage.

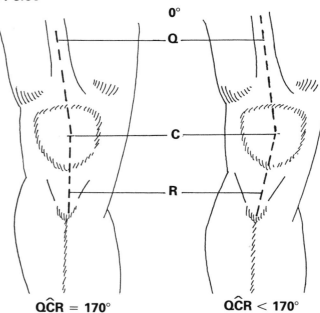

F. 5.56

QĈR = 170°   QĈR < 170°

Tibial lesions (Figure 5.59) are focused in the posterior quarter of the medial tibial condyle MTC and on the posterior margin of the medial tibial condyle PMT: the initial appearance is in the form of longitudinal streaks[82] disappearing through abrasion of the tibial condyle and the posterior margin of the medial tibial condyle.

Posterior exploration through a medial retro-ligamentous counter-incision[83] making it possible to evaluate three significant stages:

(1) In the subluxation position obtained by lateral rotation LR (Figure 5.60), tibiofemoral lesions provide a mirror image of double streaking.

(2) In the luxation position obtained by lateral hyper-rotation LHR (Figure 5.61), the extreme forward position of the tibial condyle makes it possible to observe the femoral condyle being supported by its anterior ulceration on the fractured posterior margin of the medial tibial condyle[84], while separation of the capsule-periosteum is obvious.

---

79 Destruction of the PHMM totally frees the knee for lateral rotation by eliminating the blocking effect of the meniscus (p. 47), leaving the medial tibial condyle MTC free to escape forward and possibly to become dislocated, losing all contact with the medial femoral condyle MFC.

80 Disattachment of the posterior capsule-periosteum occurs at the expense of the medial posterior capsule MPC, forming a luxation chamber occupied by the medial femoral condyle MFC.

81 The transverse streaks on the medial femoral condyle MFC are the mark of the support it has provided successively as abnormal mobility worsens and tibial condyle movement increases both forward and rearward (Figure 5.57).

82 Longitudinal streaks on the medial tibial condyle MTC are a reflection of slippage produced by successive femoral condylar support on a reduced tibial condyle surface area.

83 Anterior exploration through a medial parapatellar incision will only show femoral lesions and those only in complete flexion.

84 Fracture of the posterior margin of the medial tibial condyle PMT produces one or several microfragments, bones or osteocartilage, barely visible on the standard x-ray.

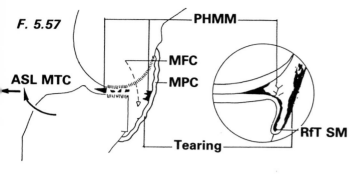

F. 5.57

ASL MTC

PHMM

MFC

MPC

RfT SM

Tearing

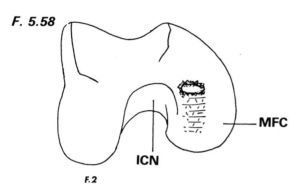

F. 5.58

MFC

ICN

F. 2

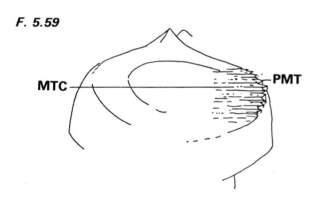

F. 5.59

MTC

PMT

(3) In the reduction position obtained through medial rotation MR (Figure 5.62), the rearward movement of the tibial condyle indicates the presence of advanced tibial lesions with the excavated tibial condyle[85] and a worn down posterior margin of the medial tibial condyle[86].

Lateral rotary instability is confined to lateral rotary dislocation. The lateral view (p. 77) can be enlarged to show modifications in the contour of the posterior part of the medial tibial condyle (Figures 5.60–5.62).

Opaque arthrography (p. 81) shows dilaceration of the posterior horn of the medial meniscus PHMM and separation of the capsule-periosteum, whose pseudodiverticular image of the posteromedial area of the tibial condyle is sometimes completed by injection of the reflected head of the semimembranous muscle RfT SM (Figure 5.57, right).

The lateral compartment
This is a complication of a ligamentous injury in medial rotation, and is less frequent and less stereotyped than that of the medial compartment: the anterolateral laxity (p. 96) is mostly involved in its global form (p. 111).

As a rule, osteocartilaginous lesions are discrete. The stellate fracture of the femoral condyle bears the mark of its contact with the dulled head of the tibial condyle.

Abnormal movement of the pivot shift is accompanied by a double hitch at the top of the tibial condyle (p. 74).

The pivot shift produces a rather vigorous response with a painful plane sign.

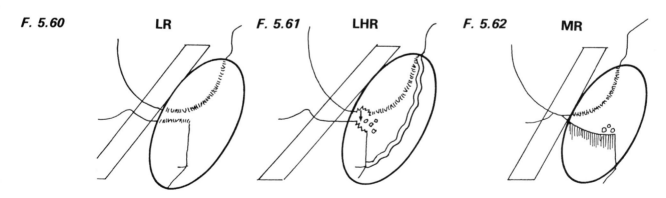

F. 5.60 LR **F. 5.61** LHR **F. 5.62** MR

---

85 The medial tibial condyle MTC is deformed in a dish-shape.

86 The posterior margin of the medial tibial condyle PMT losses its normally sharp-edged contour (p. 12), and has a blunt or eroded appearance.

Arthrosis

Arthrosis is the culmination of any chronic capsular, meniscal and ligamentous lesion of more or less short duration.

Pathogenesis
The involution of cartilage has several results. In particular highly differentiated tissues whose specialization has been attained at the cost of a certain amount of stability are predisposed to early wear[87]. Intense friction created by abnormal mobility in association with weight-bearing produces a grating effect under pressure. The synovial membrane 'tires' of fulfilling its dual function of resorption of waste resulting from wear and secretion of synovial fluid to reduce friction, etc.

With age, the cartilage's ability to adapt[88] to articular constraints (p. 52 and Note 71) gradually dwindles, and this occurs more rapidly when there is loss of stability resulting from a capsular, meniscular and ligamentous lesion.

Clinical examination
The dominant feature is pain and a decrease in the range of joint movement. The mechanical pain (p. 64) becomes more intense and sometimes more extended on the basis of how the inflammation progresses[89]. The passive limitation of joint movement (p. 70) is an overall effect, but the only handicap is the loss of complete extension[89].

Radiological examination
Arthrosis of the knee shows both general and specific symptoms.

There are three diagnostic signs which may occur separately or together: pinching of the bone interline[90], bone densification, and marginal osteophytosis[91].

A typical case is stamped with the mark of the capsular, meniscal and ligamentous lesion (Figure 5.63). Anteromedial laxity (p. 97) has osteocartilaginous complications in the medial compartment (pp. 111 and 112): the remodelling occurring in arthrosis abrades the posterior margin of the medial tibial condyle while building it up with an osteophyte. This deepens the hollowing deformation of the medial tibial condyle MTC, while the medial femoral condyle MFC loses its roundness in the support zone.

Anterolateral laxity (p. 96) has osteocartilaginous complications in the lateral compartment (p. 113): the remodelling of arthrosis transforms the lateral tibial condyle LTC into a vast dish surrounded by osteophytes. Global laxity, of whatever type, concludes in generalized arthrosis, but is nevertheless stamped with the mark of the preceding examples. The isolated lesion of the PCL (p. 100) continues through a long period of apparent improvement before terminating in classical arthrosis, nevertheless stamped with the mark of patellofemoral dominance[92].

Special examinations
Special examinations are useful at the early, or infraradiological stages of arthrosis.

Opaque arthrography (p. 81) consists of three stages:

(1) The cartilaginous stage shows the dwindling of cartilage (Figures 5.64 and 5.65): the cartilage interline CI increases in the form of a thickening of an opaque channel while the bone interline BI is maintained by the interposition of the intact or calcified meniscus.

(2) The meniscal stage reflects deterioration of the cartilage (Figure 5.66): the cartilage interline CI continues increasing, converging toward the bone interline BI, which becomes pinched through degeneration of the meniscus[93].

---

87 'Physiological' aging should be considered as a possibility from age 40.

88 The cartilage's faculty of adaptation is connected with a structure that provides it with both strength and elasticity. The strength results from a microstructure of fibrils that enable the cartilage to stand up firmly to the constraints of extended support and static effort. The elasticity is provided by a protein compound, chondroitin, which bathes the fibrils, enabling the cartilage to stretch and consequently to spread the constraints of short-term support and dynamic effort over the largest surface area.

89 Chronic irritation of the synovial membrane can be explained by the 'inflammatory' continuation of pain, and by the 'inflammatory' retraction of the capsule as the source of a forum of stiffness that is more important in flexion than in extension, because the capsule is not as lax in the rear as in the front.

90 Pinching of the interline opening corresponds to destructive arthrosis. Interline pinching may be accompanied by opening in the opposing interline; tibiofemoral interline pinching is often preceeded by 'lipping', in other words splaying of the borders in the form of lips that are moulded to the form of the meniscus once it is forced back to the border of the joint by weight-bearing.

91 Bone densification and marginal osteophytosis correspond to constructive arthrosis but follow the design of 'a blind effort at repair'. Increased density results from accumulation of new bony trabeculae under the condylar plate. They are in the centre of the support zone and are thereby crushed during weight-bearing. The osteophytosis is a reflection of an efflorescence, but is outside the support zone of the new bony trabeculae. They fill the empty space and orientate themselves in relation to traction of the capsule.

F. 5.63

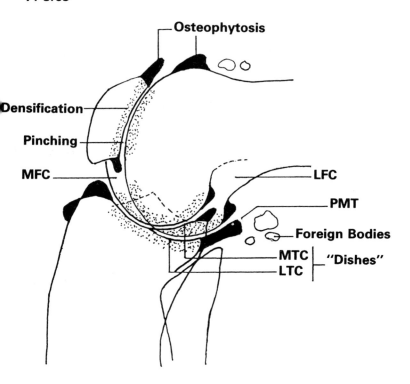

- Osteophytosis
- Densification
- Pinching
- MFC
- LFC
- PMT
- Foreign Bodies
- MTC | "Dishes"
- LTC |

F. 5.64

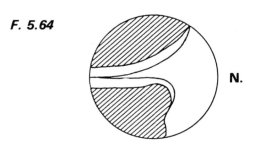

N.

F. 5.65

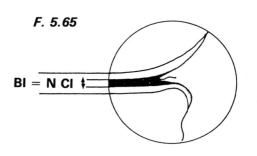

BI = N CI

F. 5.66

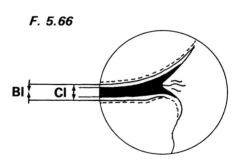

BI   CI

F. 5.67

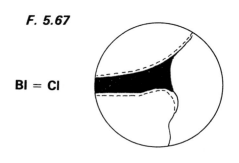

BI = CI

(3) The osseous stage confirms the destruction of the cartilage (Figure 5.67): the cartilage interline CI fuses with the bone interline BI, whose disappearance is linked to atrophy or luxation of the meniscus.

Arthroscopy (p. 84) is a useful form of exploration that is both macroscopic and microscopic (biopsy).

Course
The course can be accelerated by the appearance of a number of foreign bodies coming from secondary osteochondromatosis[94], while the very heavy handicap results mostly from ankylosis in flexion (p. 66 and Note 27).

---

92 Patellofemoral arthrosis is caused by the increase of the force of patellar compression of the femur PR: posterior subluxation of the whole tibia causes the anterior tibial tuberosity ATT to move rearward in flexion, thereby closing the lateral view of angle QCR, increasing to the same extent the force of PR considerably by using the full power of the quadriceps (p. 57).

93 Meniscal degeneration in connection with arthrosis is less stereotyped than that related to the isolated meniscal lesion (p. 90) but shows more variation: compression through flattening, blunted top, irregular sides, tibial side absent through meniscal-tibial symphysis, overall contour contracted through subluxation, etc.

94 The irritative synovitis connected with arthrosis that has become chronic results in cartilaginous metaplasia of the synovium. They produce small cartilaginous tumours: once the foreign bodies have been liberated, they increase in size and become osteocartilaginous, in other words capable of blocking knee movement and producing x-ray images of arthrophytes in the joint (Figure 5.63).

Muscular Atrophy

Muscular atrophy is the immediate reaction to the initial accident, and chronic capsular, meniscal and ligamentous lesion, become irreversible in the absence of treatment.

The pathogenesis of muscular involution brings into play a number of features, among which are:

● The defence reaction triggered by pain (p. 66).

● Immobilization imposed by incapacity or treatment.

● The relative fragility of the quadriceps[95] which 'wastes away most rapidly and takes the longest time to recover' of all muscles of the lower limb, while being the largest and most powerful.

The clinical picture is dominated by giving way[96], and assessment of the musculature (p. 69) makes it possible to evaluate the condition.

Treatment allows the course toward irreversibility to be avoided in cases of isolated lesions of the anterior cruciate ligament (p. 95 and 101) and the posterior cruciate ligament (p. 100), given the absence of a handicap, and this is true to an even greater extent in athletes with high physical capabilities.

Trophostatic syndrome
Trophostatic syndrome is the final stage of any untreated chronic lesion affecting all of the articular and periarticular structures of the knee: in fact, this chronic stage of the capsular, meniscal and ligamentous lesion is completed (p. 111) and possibly complicated (p. 112), while causing involution of both the cartilage (p. 114) and the muscles (p. 116).

Deterioration can subsequently accelerate in a vicious circle, and is exacerbated by the presence of aggravating mechanical factors. The vicious circle (Figure 5.68) reaches an end-stage consisting of arthrosis and muscle wasting. Arthrosis modifies the rolling and sliding conditions (p. 39), and muscle wasting creates joint slackness. These in their turn have repercussions on the capsular, meniscal and ligamentous lesion by increasing

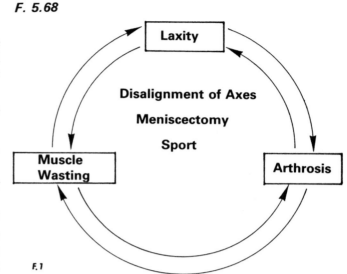

F. 5.68

abnormal mobility[97] and knocking the proprioceptive reflex system out of adjustment (p. 60 and Note 97), etc.

Aggravating mechanical factors
There is a series of three categories of aggravating mechanical factors that may activate this deterioration:

(1) Disalignment of the axes
The overload on the medial compartment in genu varum and the lateral compartment activate deterioration by creating secondary arthrosis. Genu varum, which is obvious in a frontal view (p. 65 and Note 23), is confirmed with radiological examination (p. 79) by the shift inward of the mechanical axis MA and by the increase in the tibiofemoral angle FOT (Figure 5.69). Its constitutional origin is reflected by bilateral occurrence, family and hereditary aspects, male predominance, maximum frequency in childhood and adolescence, sometimes perpetuated in the adult as a result of the moulding influence of certain sports, including soccer, with the association of a coxa vara and a pes varus. Its acquired origin is indicated by unilateral occurrence, appearing as the sequel to an impacted fracture of the medial tibial plateau, of a medial meniscectomy and pinching of the bone interline, or lateral laxity resulting from capsular, meniscal and ligamentous lesion.

Development toward arthrosis through overloading of the medial compartment may be the consequence of lateral laxity, aggravated by liberation of varus demands (p. 104 and Note 64; p. 106 and Note 72), or by medial laxity protected by release of injured medial structures.

---

95 The vastus medialis is particularly fragile, both as a recent evolutionary acquisition and because it functions both in stabilization and movement (pp. 53—60).

96 The 'giving way' is more a reflex (p. 64 and Note 17) than connected with a loss of muscle strength, and manifests itself particularly when descending stairs, which requires stabilization of the knee by the quadriceps when support is on a single foot (p. 58).

97 The axes of flexion and rotation become impossible to define.

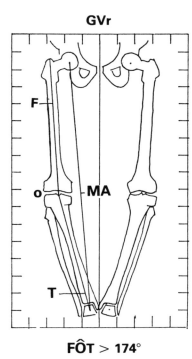

F. 5.69

GVr

FÔT > 174°

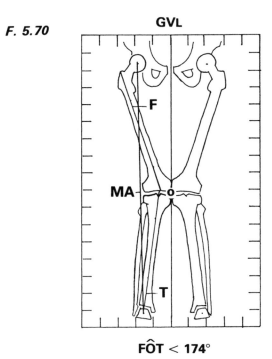

F. 5.70

GVL

FÔT < 174°

Genu valgum, which is obvious in a frontal view (p. 65 and Note 24) but obscured in obese women, is confirmed by frontal radiological examination (p. 00). Its important feature is the shift outward of the mechanical axis MA and decrease in the tibiofemoral angle FOT (Figure 5.70). Its constitutional origin is reflected in its bilateral occurrence, family and hereditary aspects, female predominance, with maximum frequency in childhood and adolescence, and minimum frequency in young adults, as well as association of a coxa valga and a pes valgus. Acquired origin is suggested by unilateral occurrence, appearing as the sequel to an impacted fracture of the lateral tibial plateau, of a lateral meniscectomy through pinching of the bone interline, or medial laxity resulting from capsular, meniscal and ligamentous lesion.

Development in the direction of arthrosis through overloading of the lateral compartment may be the consequence of poorly tolerated medial laxity, resulting from increases in the lateral resultant of lateral constraints (p. 61 and Note 99) or lateral laxity masked by relaxation of injured lateral structures.

(2) Meniscectomy
Complete ablation of the meniscus activates deterioration starting with a number of aggravating conditions, which are not only capable of combining but may potentiate one another. Disalignment of the axes (p. 116 et seq) is essentially connected with the disappearance of the meniscal wall (p. 16) and dwindling of the support zone in flexion (p. 41 and

Note 32), resulting in an increase of pressure in the corresponding compartment. Modifications in rolling/sliding (p. 39), the loss of congruity in extension (p. 35 and Note 17) and the elimination of the blocking feature of the meniscal horns (p. 42), lead to an increase in abnormal mobility.

On the whole, the increase in pressure and abnormal mobility that follow a complete meniscectomy leave the cartilaginous covering open to forceful attack[98], thereby justifying a preventive therapeutic attitude[99].

Sports

The constraints of sports, particularly high level sports, promote deterioration through demands for performance and choice of certain particular sports[100]: the threat to the cartilage is at least as serious when the knee is subjected to the disproportionate demands of a musculature that escapes wasting.

98 Direct contact of the cartilaginous surfaces produces forceful friction, particularly in free rotation where the femoral and tibial condyles are sliding in opposite directions (pp. 42 and 47), equivalent to slippage that doubles friction; the tibiofemoral articulation left fragile by the absence of the meniscal apparatus consequently shares the fate of the patellofemoral articulation (p. 35 and Note 19), which is destined for precocious arthrosis.

99 The preventive attitude toward meniscectomy means taking the maximum conservative approach: ● meniscal reinsertion in case of isolated disinsertion; ● excision of an isolated 'bucket handle'; ● abstaining in degeneration without clinical expression; and ● eventual correction of disalignment of the axis in cartilaginous lesions.

100 Soccer, rugby, hand ball, track and field events (p. 53 and Note 71) are the most destructive to cartilage: the harmful effects arise more from sudden starts and stops than from the speed of execution.

Luxation of the knee

Luxation of the knee is the 'ultimate' ligamentous injury (p. 93), terminating in dislocation through partial rupture of the capsule and ligaments.

Pàthogenesis

There are two forms.

Rotary luxation

The trigger mechanism involves no direct contact, but results from twisting of the knee with support, and a medial or lateral rotary component[101]. The capsule and ligaments are only partially ruptured sparing the menisci[102] and the peripheral structures that serve as the pivot. There is only partial dislocation with partial bone contact maintained between a tibial and femoral condyle.

Luxation in rotation O

The trigger mechanism involves direct contact, and results from forced movement of the knee in zero rotation with the heel as a support; the direct violence is anterior, with impact on the anterior tibial tuberosity[103]. There is partial rupture of the capsule and ligaments, starting with the posterior cruciate ligament and occasionally sparing the fascia lata. Dislocation is only partial, with some bone contact maintained between the posterior edge of the femoral condyles and the anterior edge of the tibial condyles.

Clinical examination

The condition is often evident. The interview indicates the violence of the initial accident; the examination is demonstrative through the extent of abnormal mobility demonstrated in extension (p. 71 et seq).

Radiological examination

This is occasionally the only determinant. Standard views are used (p. 76 et seq), looking for a juxta-articular bone fragment fracture. Reproduction of the dislocation under general anaesthesia (p. 86) under the conditions of the initial accident re-establishes the diagnosis of spontaneously reducable forms.

Course

The course depends upon vascular and nerve lesions[104].

Patellar imbalance

Patellar imbalance[105] is an anomaly in the operation of the extensor apparatus that produces a lateral shift of the patella in the frontal plane and faulty advance of the patella on the trochlea in the sagittal plane.

Patella imbalance in the frontal plane

Pathogenesis

Pathogenesis is based on an abnormal lateral position of the anterior tibial tuberosity ATT that accentuates frontal plane disalignment in extension (p. 33) and delays alignment in flexion (p. 37); abnormal mobility occurs along with morphological modifications and chronic or acute lesions. Abnormal lateral position of the anterior tibial tuberosity occurs for a number of reasons, all of which can be listed under two headings:

Static or osseous causes

In these the overly lateral position of the anterior tibial tuberosity can be combined with a more or less accentuated hyper-rotary component of the tibia:

(1) *Abnormal lateral position of the ATT in lateral tibial hypertorsion.* This is due to excess torsion of the proximal tibial metaphysis exceeding physiological tibial torsion (maximum considered

---

101 The twisting occurs when approaching extension, and is similar to that of the isolated lesion of the anterior cruciate ligament ACL variation 1 (p. 95) and anterolateral laxity (p. 96) in varus-lateral rotation, except for the abruptness of the rotary movement.

102 The line of rupture normally passes above and below the meniscal wall (p. 16).

103 Forced movement occurs in neutral flexion at 90°, and is similar to the isolated lesion of the posterior cruciate ligament (p. 100), except for the greater direct violence (Figure 5.37).

104 Vascular and nerve complications include the popliteal artery being torn loose and delaceration of the popliteal branch of the sciatic nerve, more often laterally than medially.

105 The study of patellar imbalance excludes: permanent or recurring luxation of the patella in infants; luxation of the patella in cerebral motor insufficiency; and patellofemoral arthrosis in primary gonarthrosis or secondary to disalignment in genu varum and genu valgum.

106 Lateral tibial hypertorsion frequently enters into a more complex framework, associating excess anterversion of the neck of the femur, a flat foot or a pseudo talipes canus, etc. All these anomalies integrate into the growth of the entire lower limb, which then finds the optimal adaptation necessary for standing and walking.

to be 30°) with frequent association of other anomalies of the hip and the foot[106].

(2) *Abnormal lateral position of the ATT in constitutional genu valgum.* This is caused by disalignment of the tibiofemoral axis but, as a rule, is moderate and voluntary, and associated with other causes of abnormal positioning.

(3) *Isolated abnormal lateral position of the ATT* is the most frequent. It is due less to overly lateral positioning of the ATT than to lateral hyper-rotation of the tibia under the femur[107].

Dynamic or capsular and ligamentous causes

In these, the overly lateral position of the ATT results from abnormal lateral position of the ATT in constitutional laxity; this is caused by lateral hyper-rotation in constitutional laxity, and abnormal lateral position of the ATT in acquired laxity; this is caused by lateral hyper-rotation in acquired laxity, normally anteromedial (pp. 97 and 112), originating in a lateral rotary ligamentous injury.

Abnormal mobility results in subluxation or lateral luxation[108].

The morphological modifications connected with the moulding power of growth occur particularly in isolated malposition and hypertorsion, and can take two forms.

Patellofemoral dysplasia

This is characterized by a predominance of the lateral compartment over the medial compartment[109], while maintaining a certain degree of articular congruency[110].

Distension of the soft tissues

This affects the medial stabilizers, the oblique part of the vastus medialis[111] and the medial capsular and ligamentous apparatus[112], always including involvement of the medial patellar retinaculum.

The lesions are classified in terms of the extent of abnormal mobility.

Chronic lesions occurring in lateral subluxation

A lateral compartment lesion beginning in the middle third of the support zone, subsequently spreading like an oil slick over the lateral patellar and trochlear facets, is a rapidly-developing condition, though common because it occurs regularly in arthrosis (p. 114 et seq). 'Wearing' occurs more rapidly and will result in major arthrosis[113], which is occasionally accompanied by retraction of the lateral patellar retinaculum[114].

A medial compartment lesion is circumscribed in the middle third of the support zone and undergoes little development, but is practically specific in the presence of chondromalacia[115], and passes through a series of three stages. Edematous chondromalacia, which is often difficult to recognize on the medial patellar facet by its dulled appearance and particular softness of the cartilage[116], can 'heal' spontaneously or remain undetected. Fissural chondromalacia, is easy to detect on the mediopatellar facet by fissures that continue up to the subchondral bone, and which may rapidly become fibrillar[117]. Ulcerating chondromalacia, which strips the subchondral bone of the mediopatellar facet, sometimes produces a mirror lesion on the medial trochlear facet. This actually corresponds to an extension of lateral compartment lesions above the patellar crest of the trochlear throat.

---

107 Isolated abnormal lateral position of the ATT can thus be considered as having simultaneous static and dynamic origins, in other words osseous origins, through lateral hypertorsion of the tibia and capsular and ligamentous origins through lateral hyper-rotation of the tibiofemoral joint.

108 The lateral shift of the patella is conditioned by predisposing factors (p. 53, 56 and 57). An abnormal static or dynamic position narrows the QCR angle in the frontal plane: an increase in lateral force on the patella results, and is responsible for its lateral shift to the extent that this is possible. In fact the possibilities are based on release of the medial stabilizers, particularly the oblique part of the vastus medialis, which no longer maintains its role as a guard. An abnormal dynamic position also widens the QCR angle in the sagittal plane through anterior subluxation of the tibia: the result is a decrease in the force pressing the patella on the femur, which makes a lateral shift easier from the point when the patella is disengaged.

109 The lateral shift of the patella makes greater demands on the lateral compartment than on the medial compartment, so that the medial compartment fails to develop or develops less than normal while being subjected to a relative hypopressure.

110 For the most part, articular congruency is maintained by reciprocal moulding of the patella and trochlea with the quadriceps responsible for the modelling variations of growth, except perhaps at the end of the maturation phase when different rates of maturation can occur. In fact, the false impression of 'dysplastic patella with normal trochlea' is the result of a time lag between ossification of the trochlea and the patella.

111 Distension of the oblique part of the vastus medialis (p. 23) is usually secondary. Secondary distension is the result of excess lateral demand on the patella, exceeding the recall possibilities of the oblique part of the vastus medialis. Primary distension can occur with an insertion anomaly of the patellar attachments of the oblique part of the vastus medialis.

112 Distension of the medial peripheral apparatus (p. 20) is an essential feature in dynamic causes based on constitutional and acquired laxity.

113 'Wearing' that conditions the particular functioning of the patellofemoral joint (p. 22 and Note 19, p. 24 and Note 22) is caused by hyperpressure in the lateral compartment.

114 Retraction of the lateral patellar retinaculum is primary in the permanent luxation of infancy, and is secondary here, though delayed and variable.

115 The softening is the consequence of hypopressure in the medial compartments and polymicrotraumatology due to the patella's continued attempts to recentre itself.

116 The softening produces a ping-pong-ball sensation when the cartilage is palpated with a hard instrument.

117 Fibrillar chondromalacia results in an 'unmasking' of the fibrils. They emerge from the fundamental tissue, in other words the chondroitin, the disappearance of which announces the loss of elasticity in the cartilage.

Acute lesions related to lateral luxation

Ligamentous lesions can affect the medial patellar retinaculum (p. 20) in three possible locations. Femoral disinsertion involved in anteromedial laxity (p. 97), can be difficult to distinguish from a high lesion on the tibial collateral ligament that makes up part of the same insertion on the medial epicondyle of the femur. A middle tear, which is difficult to diagram in ecchymotic tissue, will always heal spontaneously. Patellar disinsertion (the most frequent location) involves contact at the patella itself with the possibility of avulsion of bone at the moment of luxation.

Osseous lesions, in which the medial femoropatellar ligament resists or breaks, consists of four types of fracture with possible combinations. A pure chondral fracture (Figure 5.71) consists of simple lamination of the patellar crest at the top of the lateral facet of the trochlea LFT, with the medial patellar retinaculum MPR being stretched tight. A pure bone fracture (Figure 5.72) is an avulsion of

bone, as indicated above, but can be confused with the ossification that occurs during scar formation in a simple patellar disinsertion of the distended medial patellar retinaculum MPR. Osteochondral fractures (Figures 5.73 and 5.74) occur on the medial facet of the patella MFP, isolating a medial patellar fragment[118]. They affect the lateral facet of the trochlea LFT, isolating a lateral trochleocondylar fragment[119].

Clinical and radiological examination

Lateral patellar subluxation syndromes

The interview is explicit. Instability and giving way (p. 64) result from an inhibitory reflex of the muscle[120] and occur particularly when descending stairs, walking on uneven ground, and during fatigue and certain sports such as tennis, judo and the high jump, etc., with the most severe major form falling into the category of an 'articular syncope', terminating in a fall.

F. 5.71

F. 5.72

F. 5.73

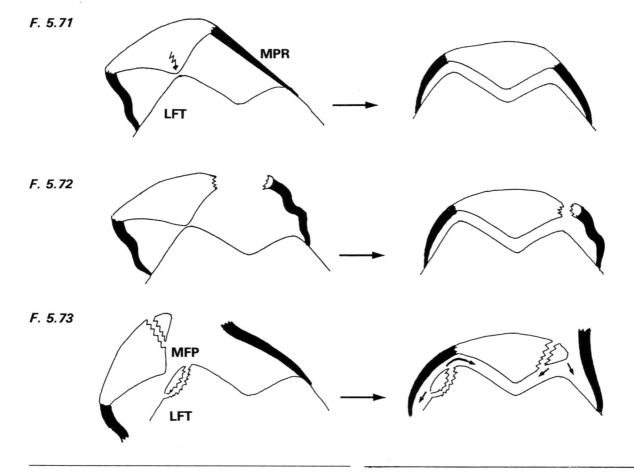

118 The medial patellar fragment may be intra-articular, and free-floating or may become para-articular by settling in the medial recess of the synovium.

119 The lateral trochleocondylar fragment undergoes the same fate as the medial patellar fragment, but with a clear predominance for exclusion from the lateral recess of the synovium.

Pain (p. 64) is suggestive: it is always vertical and may also be medial or lateral, following the margins of the patella, and triggered or aggravated by pressure, such as sitting for an extended period of time (the 'movie' sign, walking up stairs, or taking part in certain sports such as cycling, etc.). Sliding disorders (p. 64) produce signs in the sector where flexion begins, particularly in the form of pseudolocking occurring in inhibitory reflex of the muscle[120].

Clinical examination sometimes shows effusion that can be evacuated to better evaluate the objective signs. Effusion verified by patellar impact (p. 66) corresponds to mechanical hydrarthrosis (p. 76).

Patellar pain on palpation (p. 66) is reproduced in flexion with the range of movement indicating the site of the lesion (p. 67). Other signs are transverse hypermobility of the patella (p. 68) to the outside; the 'plane' sign (p. 71), usually delayed, indicating an advanced lesion; and quadriceps wasting (p. 70), which is predominant in the vastus medialis.

Radiological examination is significant in terms of axial view (p. 78).

Subluxation (Figure 5.74) is indicated by lateral overlapping of the patella[121] and by an increase in the divergence of the medial interline.

Patellofemoral dysplasia (Figure 5.75), sometimes only recognizable in the beginning, can be regarded as having five stages, beginning with a decreasing of the angle of the patella combined with an opening of the angle of the trochlea.

Stage I is the most frequent and least evident of the subnormal angles. It is identified by the narrowness of the medial facet of the patella MFC[122] and the medial facet of the trochlea MFT.

Stage II is where the patella resembles a military beret ($\hat{R} = 110°$), while the narrowing of the medial facet of the trochlea MFT increases with a relatively shallow trochlear groove.

Stage III is a semipatella on a flat trochlea ($\hat{T} = 180°$).

Stage IV shows a concave patella, like a half moon, facing a convex trochlea.

Stage V is distinctive by its large pebble-shaped patella[123] facing a similarly disproportionate trochlea.

Delayed detection of *Arthrosis* is confirmed in the lateral compartment (Figure 5.76) by three signs (p. 114), which are: pinching of the lateral interline; increased density under the lateral facet; and opposing lateral osteophytes.

Special examinations provide valuable aid in the initial or infraradiological stage. Opaque arthrography (p. 81) shows the 'pipe-shaped' deformity (Figure 5.77) with a thickened opaque channel in the medial compartment and relatively thinner one in the lateral compartment[124]. Arthroscopy (p. 84) provides a direct view.

Patellar lateral luxation syndrome
The interview is of primary importance in reconstructing the luxation and its trigger mechanism.

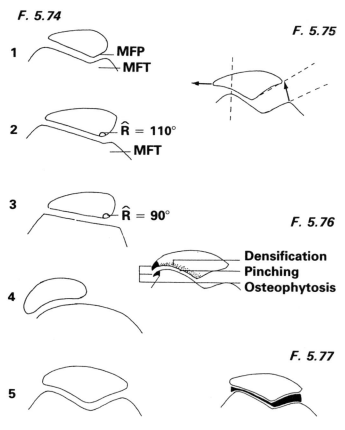

F. 5.74

1 MFP
   MFT

2 $\hat{R} = 110°$
   MFT

3 $\hat{R} = 90°$

4

5

F. 5.75

F. 5.76

Densification
Pinching
Osteophytosis

F. 5.77

---

120 The inhibitory reflex of the quadriceps muscles is equivalent to a short circuit produced by abnormal contact of articular surfaces in an area of damaged cartilage; the abnormal contact produced during movement triggers a protective reflex to avoid falling.

121 The lateral position of the patella is variable.

122 The initially concave or flat contour of the medial facet becomes distinctly convex and its roundness becomes more distinct as the condition progresses.

123 Large patella is usually congenital.

124 The divergence of the medial interline and the pinching of the lateral interline deforms the opaque channel with the possible appearance of infiltrations toward fissured and ulcerated zones.

The luxation is more or less evident[125]. The luxation related by the patient and those around him is sometimes quite explicit: the patella was seen on the lateral border of the knee or there was a 'click-clack' sound[126]. It could also have occurred years ago and passed undetected: instability and dislocation are suggestive of this, and the history can sometimes be summarized in the single concept of 'effusion of synovial fluid'.

The trigger mechanism of 'true' luxation of a patella normally in equilibrium or weakened by prior patellar imbalance involves different conditions. The contact mechanism occurs with forced movement: direct violence on a tangent with the frontal plane and a medial point of impact is most often a 'nasty' sports trauma (Figure 5.78). There is no direct contact, but twisting occurs: a jump[127] and a ligamentous injury in lateral rotation[128] frequently occur in sports.

As a rule, the clinical examination is dominated by a haemarthrosis which is abundant enough to interfere with evaluation of pain on the medial margin of the patella and interferes with attempts to reproduce abnormal mobility.

Radiological examination carried out after spontaneous reduction can confirm luxation by avulsion or ossification of the medial femoropatellar ligament and an osteochondral fracture that is recent, or is consolidated in an incorrect position[129].

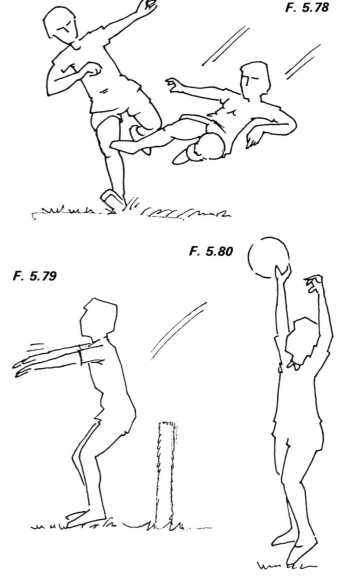

F. 5.78

F. 5.79

F. 5.80

---

125 As a rule, only the initial accident is special. Recurrence is nearly spontaneous and insidious, beginning with progressive distension of the medial dynamic mooring of the patella.

126 The audible 'click-clack' (p. 63 and Note 5) can lead to some confusion: in fact the second sound, the 'clack', indicates reduction of the luxation, sometimes giving the impression that 'the knee dislocated inward'.

127 The twisting movement of the jump described by dancers, track and field athletes, horseback riders, basketball players, etc, results in a violent contraction of the quadriceps, with the aid of a lateral rotary component that is produced on two occasions: During landing, Figure 5.79, in other words as flexion begins (p. 56) so that the patella is abruptly pressed outside of the trochlea; and during take-off, Figure 5.80, in other words at the approach to extension (p. 56) so that the patella is abruptly mobilized outside of the trochlea, with the possibility of overriding the lateral block at the extreme limit of the trochlea-femoral condyle.

128 The twisting of the lateral rotary sprain reported by the soccer player and skier at a moment of anteromedial laxity (p. 98 and Note 40) results from valgus and lateral rotation with excessive demand at the approach to extension, going beyond the elastic limit of the medial femoropatellar ligament (p. 36 and Note 21): luxation appears as a complication of a serious sprain (p. 111), but usually passing by anteromedial laxity or global anterior laxity (p. 111).

129 The radiological signs of luxation can be confused with those of subluxation (pp. 120 and 121) making up a 'background' that would more particularly indicate patellofemoral dysplasia.

Looking for the cause

Because abnormal lateral position of the anterior tibial tuberosity is recognizable by the common bayonet sign (pp. 66 and 67), it is important to specify the cause on the basis of the five possibilities mentioned above (p. 118).

The common characteristics of all osseous causes and constitutional laxity are significant: family background, bilateral occurrence, early appearance of disorders (from childhood), the aetiological or exacerbating effect of sports through polymicro-traumata (p. 87), and the frequency of morphological modifications in isolated abnormal positions of the tuberosity and in hypertorsion.

The particular characteristics that make it possible to best isolate the cause through elimination are:

Abnormal lateral position of the anterior tibial tuberosity in lateral tibia hypertorsion
This is initially recognizable in the examination and confirmed by the scanner. Clinical examination shows anomalies in support on two feet and walking (pp. 65 and 66). The deformity called pseudo-genu varum, because it can be reduced, is initially observed by convergent strabism of the patellas[130]. The increase in lumbar curvature focuses the examination on excessive anteversion of the neck of the femur accompanied by an increase in medial rotation of the hip[131]. The frequency in cases of flat foot and 'duck walk' may motivate the consultation[132].

Radiological examination is determinant in the frontal view (p. 76).

The parallel foot position (Figure 5.82) shows the femur in medial rotation MR with an enlarged image of the lateral femoral condyle LFC and a shrunken image of the medial femoral condyle MFC[133], patella shifted inwards[134], the tibia in medial rotation MR with an increase in the tibiofibular space. In the corrected foot position (Figure 5.81) with the patella brought up to its highest point, the femur recovers its normal appearance and the tibia spreads out[135] to the point of riding over the fibula.

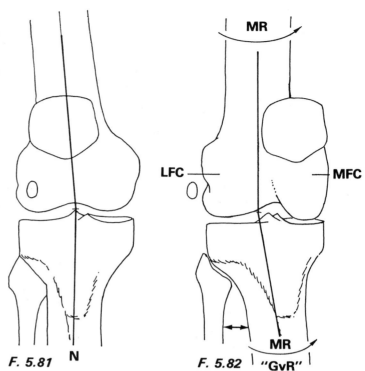

F. 5.81   N   F. 5.82   "GvR"

Tomographic CAT examination (p. 86 and Note 67) confirms hypertorsion in three sorts of combinations based on the figures obtained for the cervical-bimalleolar index[136].

The combination of lateral fibular hypertorsion and excess antevertion of the neck of the femur is the most often encountered, and it results in a slight decrease in the index to about 15°. The combination of lateral tibular hypertorsion and normal anteversion of the neck of the femur provide a moderate increase in the index to about 30°. The combination of lateral tibial hypertorsion and insufficient anterversion of the neck of the femur results in a large increase in the index to about 40°.

Abnormal lateral position of the ATT in constitutional genu valgum
Plotting of the axes (p. 78) makes it possible to positively identify constitutional genu valgum GVl (Figure 5.70).

Isolated abnormal lateral position of the ATT
Elimination of all other causes of abnormal position leads to a diagnosis of isolated abnormal position of the anterior tibial tuberosity, while noting the following features. The relative importance of the lateral hyper-rotary component of the tibia under femur in relation to the abnormal position in

---

130 The pseudo-genu varum occurring in medial rotation of osseous components while the femurs force the patellas into a 'cross-eyed' position, can be reduced by correcting foot position. The correction is aimed at bringing the patellas up to their highest point by modifying the initial parallel foot position (p. 65) by a valgus-producing lateral rotation. Reduction is complete or partial in diminishing true genu varum or in increasing true genu valgum.

131 The range of rotary movement in the coxofemoral joint, evaluated in ventral decubitus with the knee flexed at 90°, normally attains 60° in lateral rotation and 40° in medial rotation.

132 Flat feet and 'duck walk' seem to participate in the same respect as lateral tibial hypertorsion, in other words as compensating features for the hip anomaly. In fact, walking 'pigeon-toed' is nearly impossible in cases of imposed medial rotation through excess anteversion of the neck of the femur, and re-establishment of a normal step angle (p. 66 and Note 25) would be due to lateral tibial hypertorsion and possibly lateral torsion of the heel in flat feet.

133 The medial rotation MR of the femur reverses the anatomical standards for diversions of the condyles (p. 12): the medial femoral condyle MFC, whose divergence is masked, presents an in-line view. In other words it is strictly frontal with a shrunken aspect. On the other hand, the lateral femoral condyle LFC with its more apparent divergence provides a three-quarters view with an enlarged aspect.

134 The medial rotation MR of the femur forces the patella, which is linked to the trochlea, inward: the projection of the patella can brush against or ride up the medial contour of the distal end of the femur.

135 The excess of metaphyseal torsion displays the upper part of the tibia while the ankle occasionally positions itself in profile.

---

136 In reality, hypertorsion is integrated into a context that is difficult to determine when other parameters are taken into account, including talacalcanean divergence, etc.

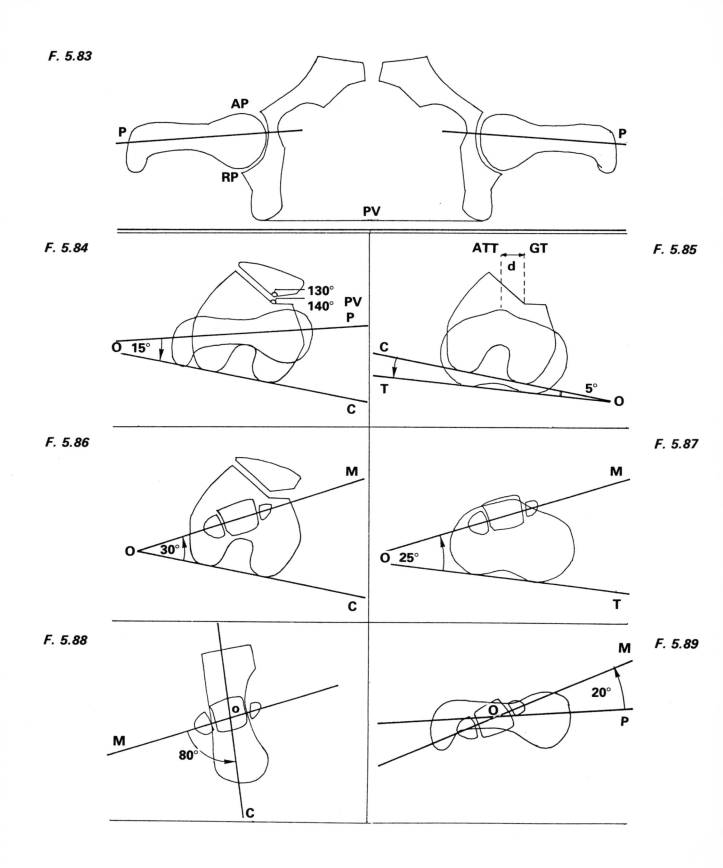

F. 5.83

F. 5.84

F. 5.85

F. 5.86

F. 5.87

F. 5.88

F. 5.89

124

hypertorsion and genu valgum; and possible hiding of the isolated bayonet sign through permanent lateral subluxation of the patella, which can give the impression of normal alignment of the extensor apparatus.

Abnormal lateral position of the ATT in constitutional laxity
Constitutional laxity 'prepares the terrain' for abnormal position, which requires the association of aggravating factors. Constitutional laxity is most often minor and is met with again in the ankles and the small distal joints[137].

Aggravating factors of the lateral shift of the patella are integrated into two types of combination; the association of constitutional laxity with a cause of osseous origin, with genu valgum GVl being the most frequently encountered; and the nearly constant association of genu recurvatum GRv[138] deceptively appears as reducible pseudo-genu varum GVr[139], but is evident in the lateral view (p. 65) and is confirmed in the radiological examination (p. 78) by a forward shift of the mechanical axis MA and by an increase in the tibiofemoral angle FOT (Figure 5.90).

F. 5.90

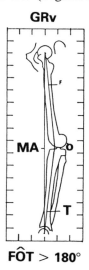

GRv

MA

FÔT > 180°

Abnormal lateral position of the ATT in acquired laxity
There is a danger of not recognizing either of these (p. 111).

Course

The course is manifested by 'crises' interspersed with more or less completely calm periods, but with the long-term result of arthrosis. The frequency of the 'crises' is influenced to an extent by five factors that somewhat precipitate the course of frontal patellar imbalance toward surgery.

Age according to three critical categories, 10 to 12 years, 16 to 20 years (period of greatest disturbance) and 30 to 40 years.

Constraints of the occupation or sport (p. 53 and Note 71) are often determinant.

Disturbing conditions: isolated lateral subluxation is both the most frequent and the most latent of complications: being aware of his abnormal knee, the individual reduces his physical activities, abandoning sports and sometimes changing his occupation. Lateral subluxation in association with lateral luxation is common and noticeable: decompensation can often be attributed to the mechanism of lateral rotary sprain[140] or damaging medial meniscectomy[141]. Pure lateral luxation is rare and not always very noticeable: as a rule, the initial accident is the only striking event[142], while recurrence occurs and nearly reduces itself spontaneously, without great disturbance.

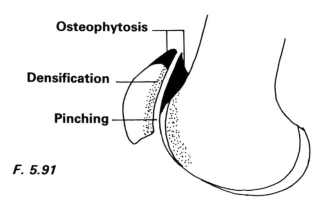

Osteophytosis

Densification

Pinching

F. 5.91

---

137 The unusual major form is singular in its generalization to a good number or all of the joints and through its characteristic appearance, particularly in the knees where lateral hyper-rotation can reach 80°.

138 Genu recurvatum GRv is manifested mostly by flattening, and at worst inverting the QCR angle in the sagittal plane (pp. 53, 56 and 57). The result is that patellar compression of the femur PC is balanced out and at worst is that it is transformed into force of anterior traction producing a 'roaming' kneecap.

139 Pseudo-genu-varum GVr, which occurs through medial rotation of the tibia under the femur, can be reduced by correcting the position of the lower limbs. The correction is aimed at obtaining a rectilinear profile for the lower limbs and thereby re-establishing 'passive' knee conditions in 0° extension, producing lateral rotation of the tibia with a valgus effect (p. 36 and 37). Reduction is total or partial, diminishing true genu varum or emphasizing true genu valgum.

140 Opposing movement of the knee in valgus-flexion/lateral rotation with support, can be sufficient without necessarily continuing into a serious sprain and to anteromedial laxity (p. 96 and 111).

141 The loss of the block formed by the posterior horn of the medial meniscus (p. 44) and possibly post-operative muscle wasting are *a priori* sufficient.

142 The initial reduction of luxation can be obtained by gentle extension so that the release of the quadriceps causes the patella to shift back into the subtrochlear groove (p. 33).

Patellofemoral dysplasia occurs, and its influence is directly proportional to the stage of advancement.

Dynamic causes that reflect the importance of the capsular and ligamentous apparatus in patellar stability. The inexorable march toward arthrosis distinguishes the course of the frontal patellar imbalance that escapes surgery (Figure 5.90)[143].

Patellar imbalance in the sagittal plane

The advance of the patella on the trochlea may be insufficient during three stages: engagement, above 30° and above 90°.

Patellar imbalance during engagement

Pathogenesis

The pathogenesis is based on an abnormally high position of the patella causing a trochleopatellar conflict with morphological modifications and chronic lesions. An overly high position of the patella in the supratrochlear fossa during extension (Figures 5.94) defines patella alta [144] in relation to the biomechanical conditions of the 'passive' (p. 32) and 'active' (p. 53) knee.

The conflict between the upper margin of the trochlea and the lower edge of the articular surface of the patella is produced as soon as flexion is initiated, in other words as soon as the patella approaches the trochlea in order for its lower third to be engaged (p. 34).

The morphological modifications linked to the moulding power of growth may occur at two levels. Excessive raising of the upper border of the trochlea, which is clearly marked on the medial facet (Figure 5.91) in relation to anatomical conditions (p. 12 and Note 4). The possible appearance of a depression of the patella at the lower part of the inferior third of its articular surface (Figure 5.94).

---

143 The singular characteristic of patellofemoral arthrosis is in the stage confirmed by a 'double walled' image (Figure 5.90): this is an osteophytic leaf that extends the trochlear groove and fills the supratrochlear fossa at an angle that approximately corresponds to the loss of extension.

144 Patella alta results from an increase in the length of the patellar tendon in relation to the height of the trochlea: the increase in length is real in terms of a normal trochlea and relative in relation to a trochlea that is reduced in height.

F. 5.92

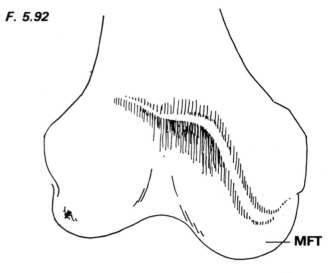

MFT

F. 5.93

F. 5.94

30°

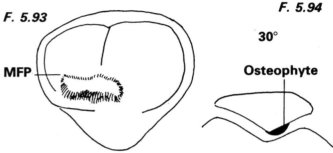

MFP

Osteophyte

F. 5.95

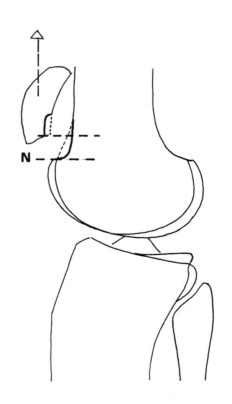

N

The chronic lesions recall fissural and ulcerating chondromalacia (p. 118), but of a particular type. The fissures that streak the top to bottom of the groove and medial facet of the trochlea MFT have a 'combed' appearance (Figure 5.91); the ulcerations cutting into the crest and lower part of the medial facet of the patella MFP announce arthrosis (Figure 5.92).

Clinical examination

The interview should reveal a history of giving way and pseudolocking (p. 119 and Note 110), with the emphasis placed particularly on the moment of landing after jumping[145]. The examination is determinant, with active mobilization reproducing the pathognomonic sign of a hitch as soon as flexion is initiated (p. 68), and occasional association with a painful jerk (p. 64 and Note 15).

Radiological examination
The standard lateral view (p. 76) occasionally shows step formation of the transition area between the supratrochlear fossa and the trochlea (Figure 5.93). An additional lateral view in extension (p. 80) makes it possible to catch the patella in an overly high position (Figure 5.94), both with and without voluntary contraction of the quadriceps[146].

Spontaneous course
The condition culminates in patellofemoral arthrosis with lower pole dominance.

Patellar imbalance beyond 30°

Pathogenesis
The pathogenesis is an improperly formed trochlea that reduces trochleopatellar support, with morphological modifications and chronic lesions. The trochlea is abnormally prominent, forming a dome[147] on which the patella rocks back and forth like a plank on a wave (Figure 5.95). The reduced support considerably increases unit pressure, resulting in a nearly linear distribution.

The morphological modifications linked to the moulding power of growth primarily affect the articular surface of the patella, with the edge of the

---

145 Twisting during landing after a jump (p. 119 and Note 117), involving a violent contraction of the quadriceps, will press the patella abruptly against the trochlea further aggravating the conflict.

146 The lower limit of the articular surface of the patella overrides the upper border of the trochlea in both cases. The x-ray in contraction serves as an additional verification.

147 The defective form can also be demonstrated in the sagittal plane, assimilating the two trochlear facets in a single double spiral whose respective radii remain abnormally small (p. 12).

F. 5.96

F. 5.97

"Pitching"

F. 5.98

F. 5.99

90°

Osteophyte

inferior third to the middle third raised in an additional crest (Figure 5.96); a pitching crest perpendicular to the vertical crest of the patella (p. 12) sometimes marks its imprint on the trochlea, forming a transverse groove.

The chronic lesions recall the three stages of chondromalacia circumscribed in the middle third of the patella (p. 118).

Clinical examination
The interview is orientated to the single concept of pseudolocking (p. 119 and Note 110). The examination may reveal the rocking patella in lateral view just beyond 30° flexion.

Radiological examination
The standard lateral view (p. 77) shows obvious sagittal dysplasia of the trochlea (Figure 5.97). The standard axial view at 30° (p. 78) is used to determine any pinching of the bone interline that would indicate arthrosis.

Spontaneous course
The path of the disease leads toward patellofemoral arthrosis, which is rare in the early stages.

Patellar imbalance beyond 90°

Pathogenesis
The pathogenesis consists of lower medial pole osteophytosis of the patella in a conflict between the condyle and patella that results in chronic lesions. The 'aggressive' patellar growth strikes the nonsupporting articular surface of the medial femoral condyle when the knee is flexed beyond 90°. Constructive lesions on the patella are destructive along the part of the medial condylar border that is continuous with the intercondylar notch.

Clinical examination
The clinical examination is similar to a pseudosyndrome of the anterior horn of the medial meniscus.

Radiological examination
The standard axial view at 90° (p. 78) may catch the patellar osteophyte 'in the act' of compression (Figure 5.98).

Spontaneous course
The disease is astonishingly static.[148].

Post-traumatic chondromalacia of the patella

The 'scoring' of patellofemoral cartilage may be partly caused by a contusion of the patella when it is serving as a 'shield'.

Pathogenesis
The topographical distribution suggests a trauma directed toward the patella. The trigger mechanism involves contact direct violence, with impact on the anterior aspects of the patella. This is essentially a patella-type lesion with a stamped-out section: the patellar cartilage appears regularly depressed, as if it were 'smashed into' the hard surface of the trochlea.

Clinical examination
The interview indicates a history of a 'swollen knee' relating to direct violence to the patella with an anterior point of impact, and possibly effusion that was aspirated (p. 81)

Examination is relatively unproductive with the exception of sensitivity of the articular surfaces reproduced by patellar palpation (p. 66) and by active mobilization while pressing the patella against the femur (p. 68).

Radiological examination
No abnormalities are seen on x-ray.

Course
The course follows one of the three stages of chondromalacia (p. 118): oedematous chondromalacia may 'heal' spontaneously in the absence of patellar imbalance, and fissular and possibly ulcerating chondromalacia with a mirror lesion is generally confirmed after a period of six months in patellar imbalance.

Post-traumatic osteochondral lesions

The destruction of cartilage down to the bone is of importance in traumatology because of its frequency and its prognosis.

Frequency of osteochondral lesions

The frequency of osteochondral lesions is too often underestimated. Lesions of the patellofemoral joint are reflected in patellar imbalance in the frontal plane (p. 118) and the sagittal plane (p. 126 et seq). Tibiofemoral joint lesions vary depending on whether or not laxity exists. (a) In the presence of laxity, medial compartment (p. 111) and lateral compartment (p. 112) lesions are tibiofemoral and most often peripheral. (b) In the absence of laxity, lesions are basically femoral and most often central. The osteochondral fracture that affects the 'wearing surface' of the medial femoral condyle arises from twisting of the knee in valgus-medial rotation with support. In other words, this is normal for a lateral rotary sprain without causing it[149].

Spectacular locking results during the phase when the arthrophyte is free to circulate as a loose body in the joint. X-rays clearly show the sheared medial femoral condyle, using a frontal view of the support zone and a lateral view of the anterior part of the spiral. The chondral fracture affecting the 'wearing surface' of the lateral femoral condyle arises from twisting the knee in a position of varus-medial

---

148 The condylar and patellar conflict have an extremely limited development, which is most often discovered during an operation.

149 Twisting (p. 98 and Notes 39 and 40) is produced when the knee is nearly extended, which reduces the risk of abnormal mobility: the meniscal, capsular and ligamentous apparatus can therefore resist, but at the cost of shearing off the medial femoral condyle, which is held in place by the particular shape of the medial compartment.

rotation with support. In otherwords this is normal for a medial rotary sprain without causing it[150]; flaking of the anterior part of lateral femoral condyle cartilage is most often discovered during an operation.

The chondral fracture affecting the open areas of the femoral condyles arises from a forced movement of the knee caused by direct violence with anterior or lateral impact, in other words normal for a sprain in extension but without causing it[151]: the flaking of condylar cartilage looks like a radiating or stellate crater. The fracture, which may be a surprise discovered during an operation, cuts the medial tibial condyle at the posterior margin, notching the trochlear groove or furrowing the trochlear facet, etc.

Prognosis of osteochondral lesions

The prognosis is always reserved: osteochondral lesions create a situation predisposed to arthrosis and may precipitate the development of arthrosis (p. 84), with attempted repairs producing uncertain results[152].

Osteonecrosis

Osteonecrosis is considered to be aseptic[153] and idiopathic[154].

Pathogenesis of osteonecrosis

The pathogenesis is common to all of the various sites of involvement where vascular insufficiency modifies the mechanical resistance of the bone.

Vascular insufficiency, which undoubtedly reduces the extensibility of vascular spaces developed within bone tissue, will be triggered or aggravated by polymicrotraumatology, particularly that connected with sports (p. 87).

There are three stages in the modification of mechanical resistance in the bone: destruction, equivalent to an infarctus of the bone trabeculae[155]; reconstruction from living bone tissue around the necrosis[156] terminates, in principle, by a generally long but integral restitution, taking months and sometimes years.

Tissue healing may end up complete or incomplete. A complete cure can take place without loss of bone matter in the presence of a small necrotic fragment largely surrounded by living tissue. Incomplete healing may ensue in the presence of a large necrotic fragment that exceeds the regeneration possibilities of the living tissue. This will result in a deformity of the bone structure that can compromise the integrity of the neighbouring joint; although the knee is only slightly incapacitated in terms of the many demands made on it (including muscular contraction and weight-bearing) during this long regeneration phase, a loss of articular congruity will result, making itself felt over the long term through secondary arthrosis[157].

Symptomatology and course of osteonecrosis

The symptomatology and course are based on the various sites of involvement, with some relationship to age.

Osteonecrosis of the tibial tubercule[158]

This is a disorder of adolescence: the necrosis simultaneously attacks the two centres of ossification on the tibial tubercule, including

---

150 Twisting (p. 95 and Notes 25 and 26) is produced under the same conditions, in other words at near extension, which reduces the risk of abnormal mobility; the meniscal, capsular and ligamentous apparatus can therefore resist, but at the cost of lacerating the lateral femoral condyle which is freed by the particular shape of the lateral compartment (p. 37).

151 The forced movement can occur in flexion with neutral rotation (p. 100) as well as in extension (p. 10 et seq), but without the required conditions of support or countersupport that could result in a sprain.

152 Curettage of bone ends, and particularly perforations through the bone, may relieve pain by improving local circulatory conditions, but these measures cannot reconstitute cartilage covering. In fact, new cartilage is formed at the expense of conjunctive tissue invading the joint through the perforations and does not have the mechanical properties of strength and elasticity (p. 114 and Note 88).

153 The term 'aseptic necrosis' is used to exclude osteonecroses arising from bone infections.

154 The term 'idiopathic necrosis' is used to exclude osteonecroses of the knee that arise from known causes: fracture and luxations that belong to the category of major traumata, and osteonecrosis in elderly people, which could be considered idiopathic, but which is excluded here by definition.

155 The anatomopathological aspect of the necrosis is recognized by an essential sign: disappearance of osteocytes while cavities that contain osteocytes become 'empty tombs'.

156 The histopathological aspect of regeneration is demonstrated by the invasion of granular tissue which acts both as an agent for resorption and osteogenesis: there is simultaneous resorption of necrotic tissue and its replacement by newly formed tissue.

157 Involvement of the cartilage, a fundamental feature in secondary arthrosis (p. 87), will not be directly connected with the necrosis of bone structure: in fact, the cartilage does not have blood vessels but is basically nourished by imbibing synovial fluid, thereby maintaining its vitality, as can be seen in its normal macroscopic appearance during arthrotomy and arthroscopy.

158 Osteonecrosis of the tibial tubercule is known under other names: Osgood-Schlatter disease, osteochondritis of the tibial tubercule, anterior tibial apophysis, anterior tibial osteochondrosis.

ossification intended for the anterior tibial tuberosity ATT[159].

Clinical examination
The interview is significant in the fact that sports seem to be the cause: this disorder is practically limited to adolescent boys. The complaint involves both knees, at the same time or one after the other. As a rule, anterior pain is moderate but returns or is made worse by kneeling, descending stairs, jumping, etc, to the point of inhibiting athletic activities.

The examination reveals a normal joint and an inflammatory reaction that may reach the patellar tendon: there is sharp pain in the ATT, with tumefaction, occasionally accompanied by heat and redness.

Radiological examination
Standard views offer normal and comparative pictures. Only the lateral view can reveal a hypertrophied tubercule with an irregular and indistinct contour, but particularly fragmented into a number of bone nucleii that differ in size, shape and opacity (Figure 5.100).

Course
A complete cure can take a long time when it is not possible to impose rest, including temporary abstention from sports.

Formation of a bony nucleus in the tendon may present problems and lead to surgical excision[160].

Patellar osteonecrosis

This is a disorder of late childhood and adolescence: the necrosis separately attacks the two centres of ossification on the patella, thereby arriving in separate stages[161].

The clinical verdict on a painful knee that has no obvious cause is too often 'normal growing pains' in children who are in fact over-extended in sports during late childhood and adolescence.

Radiological examination with lateral views reveals a patella that is often reduced, in pieces or

heterogenous, with an irregular and indistinct contour.

The disease remits spontaneously.

F. 5.100

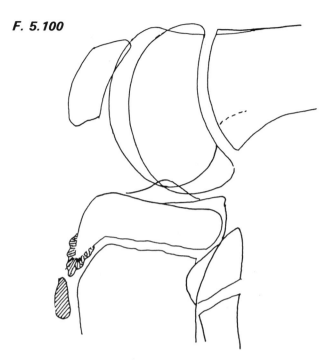

Condylar osteonecrosis

There are two distinct forms, diffuse and circumscribed.

Diffuse condylar osteonecrosis

The diffuse form is a disorder of childhood. If no biopsy has been carried out and necrosis has not been established histologically, the problem may be an ossification disorder affecting the ossification centre of one or two condyles[162].

Clinical examination
The connection with sports is that almost all patients are boys, complaining of pain in one or both knees: as a rule, this lateral pain is moderate and mechanical in its cycles, possibly becoming acute, with limping and nocturnal discomfort, leading to voluntary interruption of sports.

Examination reveals pain in the supporting surface of the condyle and particularly by the

---

159 The tibial tubercule, a sort of cartilaginous beak on the superior tibial epiphysis and directed downward and forward, contains two centres of ossification: a main centre and an accessory centre at the top of the tubercule, which appear at puberty and subsequently unite, with the diaphysis giving rise to the ATT. These undergo ossification, terminating between age 16 and 20.

160 The anato-pathology can therefore establish that necrosis exists, when it is not possible to have a complete study of the tubercule in the initial stage.

161 The patella has two centres of ossification: a main centre appearing in late childhood and a secondary centre appearing in adolescence.

162 'Diffuse condylar osteonecrosis', which is also called polymicro-osteochondritis and polymicroosteochondronecrosis, currently deserves the more appropriate term of polyosteochondrosis of the femoral condyles: endochondral ossification disorders involve a number of secondary ossification centres in the lower femoral ephiphysis.

130

pathognomonic sign of painful extension with countersupport. The child lies on his back with the knee and hip flexed at 90° and the examiner applies countersupport to the sole of the foot using his hand or shoulder. This position can vigorously counteract active distension and make it possible to note the angle of the knee in relation to the appearance of the pain[163].

F. 5.101

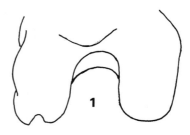

Radiological examination
Standard views are sufficiently descriptive, particularly in terms of the intercondylar notches. The seat of this single or multiple lesion is always located in the support zone of the condyle, producing any of five types of picture[164] (Figure 5.101): a simple gap (A), a gap surrounded by a dense margin (B), a gap with an irregular contour (C), a gap partially filled with an incongruent bone nucleus (D) or a congruent bone nucleus (E).

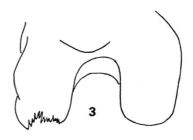

The lesion may be unilateral with involvement of one or both condyles, or bilateral with involvement of three or four condyles[165].

Tomography reveals more precise images.

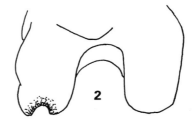

Course
Complete healing always occurs spontaneously over a more or less long term. Radiological normalization occurs when the gap is in-filled from the bottom or if the bone nucleus is reattached, progressively increasing in volume[166], though at the price of losing the roundness of the condylar contour.

Circumscribed condylar osteonecrosis

The circumscribed form is a disorder of adolescents and young adults[167]. The necrosis[168] is limited to the medial femoral condyle MFC across from the intercondylar notch ICN and isolated by 'dissection'. The necrotic fragment subsequently circumscribed

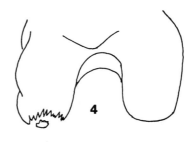

---

163 The manoeuvre used is valuable not only in diagnostic terms, but also as therapy in case of immobilization in a plaster cast. It should be carried out in a painless position: contact with the articular surfaces in the injured zone can be avoided.

164 The variety of pictures is due to different ages of lesions.

165 Radiological and clinical results may be correlated, but sometimes only on a single condyle, which poses the problem of asymptomatic pictures: in such a case would it be a subclinical stage beginning with a simple gap? or normal pictures reflecting physiological variations in epiphyseal maturation?

166 The cyclic development of ossification disorders never arrives at a phase of major destruction: in fact, the bone nucleus does not detach and become a foreign intra-articular body as occurs in dissecting osteochondritis.

167 Circumscribed osteonecrosis of the medial femoral condyle is known under other names: Koenig's disease, dissecting osteochondritis, dissecting aseptic osteonecrosis.

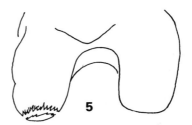

forms an element which is sequestered in a sort of 'lodging'; however, it may separate, becoming a loose body and falling into the joint[169].

Clinical examination
During the loose body phase in an adolescent or a young adult participating in sports, the interview reveals explicit findings: i.e. sliding defects (p. 64), becoming nearly pathognomonic despite the absence of prior history.

The examination is occasionally demonstrative after aspiration to evacuate hydarthrosis; the squatting test with support can cause pain, and it is occasionally possible to palpate the loose body in one of the joint pouches.

Radiological examination
Standard x-ray views provide an easy means diagnosis[170], particularly the view of the intercondylar notches showing two aspects of the

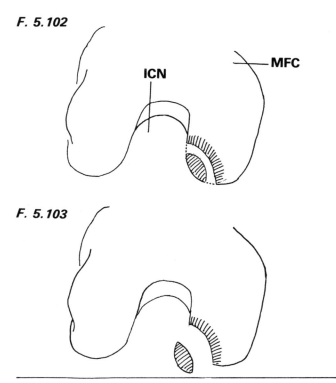

F. 5.102

ICN

MFC

F. 5.103

lesion against the lateral border of the medial condyle. The sequestered fragment is 'lodged' (Figure 5.102) sometimes with greater or lesser opacity or stippled in relation to neighbouring bone and is clearly delimited by a convex, radiotransparent line of demarcation. The loose body (Figure 5.105) is nummular or disc-shaped and sometimes larger than its notch of origin[171].

Tomography still provides the best diagnostic pictures.

Course
A complete cure is rarely obtained spontaneously. The surgical approach of ablation of the loose body, or possible fixation of the sequestered fragment, makes it possible to determine the possibility of arthrosis.

'Locking' of the proximal tibiofibular joint

Pathogenesis
Disorders of the proximal tibiofibular joint (p. 13) are infrequently diagnosed because they are poorly understood. They are a product of the polymicrotraumata to which athletes are susceptible (p. 87).

Clinical examination
Clinical examination can be summarized as revealing lateral pain of the knee descending the anterolateral area of the leg, occasionally simulating arteritis but continuing when the subject has stopped moving and abating only after support is removed. The true origin is revealed by a meticulous search for elective pain and abnormal mobility.

Elective pain is sharp on the upper tibiofibular interline, with pressure causing pain to radiate through the anterolateral area. Abnormal mobility in the sagittal plane and anterior or posterior subluxation is accompanied by a revival of elective pain and terminates in 'locking'[172].

Radiological examination
The radiographical appearance of the proximal tibiofibular channel is normal.

---

168 Confirmation is always made by surgery and possibly through histological examination.

169 There is little or no possibility of reuniting the sequestered fragment with living tissue, as happens at other sites of osteonecrosis: the cartilaginous cover, which is intact at the beginning because it is preserved by its nutritive independence, is destroyed over the edge of the necrotic fragment and subsequently opens freeing the foreign body, which may be pediculated, free or have secondary synovial attachments.

170 The pitfall of delayed x-ray image can be overcome by scintigraphy (p. 86): the hyperactive focus is significant, looking like a 'carie' that is almost imperceptibly small but is surrounded by living tissue.

171 The notch is slowly filled in while the loose body, which has one facet covered with cartilage, may continue to develop, feeding on synovial fluid.

172 The locking probably reflects anterior or posterior luxation and may be followed by release with a jerk.

Course
Spectacular remission can be obtained with infiltration corticoid therapy, which is a test that is both diagnostic and therapeutic.

Bursitis

All serous bursae [173] may be sites of inflammatory reaction that are part of occupational and sports polymicrotraumas (p. 87). There are two varieties, superficial and deep.

Superficial bursitis

Pathogenesis
The lesion is, in principle, limited to the anterior facet of the knee, which is both the most highly exposed and the best covered with serous bursae, including three prepatellar and one pretibial bursa (p. 24) that do not communicate with the joint cavity.

The trigger mechanism is usually polymicro-traumatous of the worker, traditionally a nun who is required to genuflect or kneel for extended periods of time.

The inflammatory aseptic lesion which results is the chronic or subacute type that terminates in thickening of the bursa wall [174].

Clinical examination
The clinical findings are significant because they must determine the appearance and location of the hygroma [175]. The inflammatory appearance of the hygroma is a combination of swelling, redness, heat and pain. The prepatellar and pretibial distribution of the hygroma is caused by one or both knees bearing on the ground.

Radiological examination
The lateral view may reveal 'stones of piety' consisting of calcified hygromas.

Aspiration
A fluid containing sediment may be recovered (p. 81).

Course
The condition often requires surgical drainage of the bursa.

Deep bursitis

Pathogenesis
The site of involvement is limited to the posterior facet of the knee, where the serous bursa of the popliteal tendon (p. 30), the medial head of the gastrocnemius muscle bursa (p. 20) and the gastrocnemio-semimembranous bursa (p. 20) connect with the popliteal fossa while communicating with the joint cavity.

The trigger mechanism can be attributed to occupational and sports polymicrotraumas, and generally involving a previously defect [176] and repeated or extended squatting [177]. A chronic or subacute type of inflammatory lesion occurs, characteristic of bursitis, or there may be an acute lesion such as perforation of the capsule [178], terminating in cyst formation. [179].

Clinical signs and radiological examination
True bursitis can be obvious or disconcerting on examination. The direct signs are evident in the popliteal fossa (p. 66), with deep and painful swelling of variable volume and consistency, partially connected with diffuse swelling and decreased range of knee joint movement.

Deceptive indirect signs can occur at some distance from the popliteal fossa, demonstrating nerve, artery or vein compression. Sciatica with Laseque's sign [180] may occur, but is atypical because it is more painful when walking than when standing or sitting for an extended period, and there is no spinal syndrome and no bell sign. There is intermittent claudication simulating arteritis, though walking rhythm and biological features are normal. There are also return circulation difficulties, with distal oedema and local

---

173 The serous bursae, accessories to the tendons and aponeuroses, play the role of a reflection pulley that aids sliding.

174 The thickening of the bursa wall is caused by fibrosis resulting in recurring inflammatory episodes.

175 The subcutaneous hygroma is one sort of superficial expression of chronic bursitis.

176 Prior joint defects, whether mechanical, degenerative or a malformation, are a source of generalized effusion.

177 Squatting makes it possible for the fluid to enter the gastrocnemio-semimembranous bursa via two mechanisms, mechanisms which are only possible in flexion: opening the communication with the medial gastrocnemius bursa (p. 20) and driving the effusions to the rear through intra-articular hyperpression formed by the increase in compression of the patella on the femur (p. 56).

178 Perforation of the capsule is focused on weak points and benefits from a sudden increase in intra-articular hyperpressure during a sudden squatting movement.

179 The cyst, which is more often false than true, beginning with draining of the effusion into numerous cleavage planes of the soft tissue, is a complication of bursitis by perforation.

180 Laseque's sign results from tension of the sciatic nerve caused by popliteal swelling acting as a sawhorse.

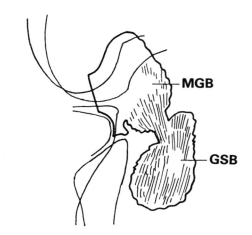

MGB

GSB

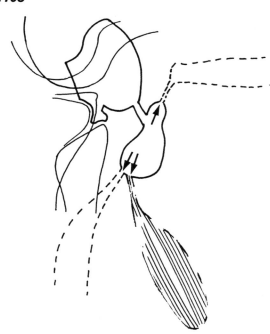

pallor, soft and pitting, which are at their worst at the end of the day.

Arthrography (p. 81) with lateral view in flexion shows that the medial head of the gastrocnemius muscle bursa and the gastrocnemio-semimembranous bursa have extended, heterogeneous and irregular areas of projection (Figure 5.104).

The 'cyst' examination findings can be deceptive at the level of the calf, which may become painful and swollen simulating thrombosis of a deep vein in the leg, but without hardening of the funiculi, and without tachycardia or fever.

Arthrography (p. 81), with lateral view in flexion, shows that the opaque liquid forms a considerable pool that tends to descend rather than ascend[181], with a penniform appearance suggestive of a rupture (Figure 5.105).

Course

The course depends on the treatment of the intra-articular deterioration; direct surgical treatment is unsuitable[182].

'Fabellitis'

The fabella, a true 'knot' (Figure 5.106) where at least three ligaments terminate and which supports the lateral head of the gastrocnemius tendon (p. 26 and Note 25), may be the cause of isolated pain in the posterolateral region of the knee resulting from the polymicrotraumata of sports (p. 89).

Pathogenesis

The pathogenesis is based on functional over-exertion of the lateral head of the gastrocnemius, which participates in a number of actions by means of the fabella, of which the two most important are: mobilizing muscular force in initiating flexion (p. 56), and serving as a driving force in necessary lateral rotation when approaching extension (p. 57 and Note 86).

Clinical examination

The interview reveals the gradual development of posterolateral pain radiating downward in the cutaneous areas served by the common peroneal nerve[183], the pain is usually moderate and related to movement (p. 64), exacerbated by muscular stretching in forced extension or by compression of the popliteal fossa when the legs are crossed.

Examination should consist of palpation in flexion and dorsal decubitus (p. 66): the acutely painful abarticular point is located in the lateral part of the popliteal fossa and clearly above the interline. Pressure on this point reproduces the radiation of sciatic pain, and occasionally the examiner can feel a hardened structure corresponding to the fabella.

---

181 The lateral view should be carried out on large format film.

182 The direct surgical approach is only suitable for non-trauma lesions, for example polyarthritis, or inflammatory synovitis proliferating from diverticular bursitis and forming a true popliteal cyst.

183 The fabella can directly compress the common peroneal nerve: radiation of pain toward the lower leg can also occur in the posterior area along its lateral (tibial) part as well as in the upper anterolateral and lower tibial parts.

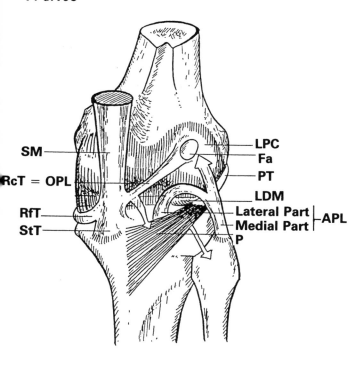

SM —
RcT = OPL —
RfT —
StT —

LPC
Fa
PT
LDM
Lateral Part ⎤
Medial Part ⎦ APL
P

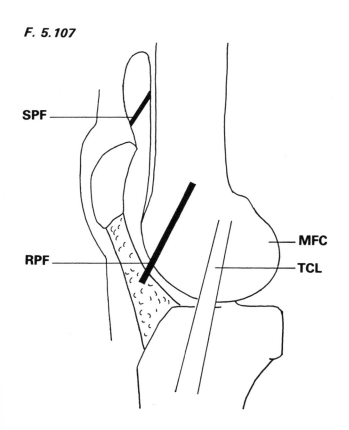

SPF —

RPF —

MFC
TCL

Radiological examination
X-ray shows the ossified fabella[184], visible in the frontal view (p. 76 and Note 49) and particularly in lateral views (p. 77).

Course
The pain may be obstinate and resistant, handicapping the athlete, with the danger of confusing the diagnosis[185].

Plica ('shelf' or fold formation)

Any synovial fold may have intra-articular repercussions, particularly through the polymicro-traumata of sports (p. 89): this is an infrequent complication, and one that is little known and poorly systematized. It consists of two sites of involvement with two anatomical entities (p. 14 and Note 9; p. 22 and Note 19).

Suprapatellar fold SPF syndrome (Figure 5.107)

Pathogenesis
The pathogenesis points to the polymicro-traumatology of sports, but on the basis of a total separation between the bursa and the pouch.

Clinical examination
The clinical examination reveals an increase in the circumscribed volume of the subquadricipital serous bursa; the normally tight and only slightly painful bulging contrasts with its crescent-shaped swelling (concave side downward) above the patella. There is disappearance of the lateropatellar hollows (p. 66) without patellar impact (p. 68).

Special examinations should include:

● aspiration of the joint, which produces a white fluid, whereas aspiration of the bursa shows hydarthrosis with sediment (p. 76).

Radiological examination
Arthrography (p. 81) shows that the contrast fluid fills the anterior pouch but can go no higher (Figure 5.108). Arthroscopy (p. 84) provides a direct view with the possibility of resection of the separation.

---

184 The fabella in its fibrocartilaginous form (p. 26 and Note 25) is radiotransparent, which means that a diagnosis of 'fabellitis' should be excluded.

185 The handicap in a high level athlete may justify excision of the fabella, provided that there is no clinical indication of a trauma-induced lateral meniscectomy.

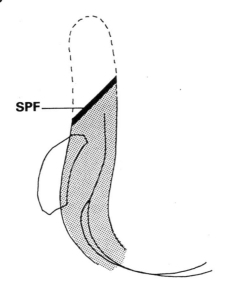

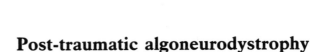

Course

The course, which is sometimes complicated by the association of patellar chondromalacia, is set on the path of a cure by simple resection of the plica.

Retropatellar fold RPF syndrome (Figure 5.107)

Pathogenesis

The pathogenesis points to polymicrotraumata in transforming the plica into a fibrous band that rubs against the medial facet of the trochlea and the medial femoral condyle like a windshield wiper.

Clinical examination

The clinical examination is summarized by isolated medial pain or the same associated with a jerk, sometimes revealed by palpation during passive movement, but accompanied by a lateral rotary component[186].

Arthrography

Special examinations should include: mixed arthrography (p. 81), using an axial view at 90°, which reveals the synovial fold (Figure 5.109); and arthroscopy (p. 84), which assesses the plica and makes resection possible.

Course

Healing results from resection of the plica, with possible persistence of a cartilaginous lesion produced by the 'windshield wiper' effect.

186 The lateral rotary component makes it easier for the jerk to appear by placing the plica under peak tension with the medial femoral condyle playing the role of a sawhorse, and palpating for a rigid cord (p. 66).

Post-traumatic algoneurodystrophy

Any trauma, even apparently mild, may result in autonomic nervous system disorders: post-traumatic algoneurodystrophy[187] nearly exclusively occurs in the knees[188] of adults over 30.

Pathogenesis

The site of involvement covers the whole knee with unilateral and single focus involvement, exceptionally with bilateral and multifocus involvement.

The trigger mechanism is local or distant trauma, mild or violent, sometimes commonplace in the form of a simple contusion or sore, possibly iatrogenic resulting from unsuitable rehabilitation or immobilization[189], etc.

Autonomic nervous system disorders remain mysterious[190], even though it is possible to suggest numerous factors favouring the condition, including psychological factors[191] and the work-related polymicrotraumata (p. 89).

187 Post-traumatic algoneurodystrophy is cited under other names: Sudeck's disease, post-traumatic bone atrophy, painful post-traumatic osteoporosis, post-traumatic neurotrophic syndrome, Leriche's disease.

188 Localized pagetoid modifications of dramatic origin, post-traumatic osteosclerosis and post-traumatic osteolysis are unusual and occur far from the knee, affecting the tibial diaphysis more often than the femoral, in other words the one with the least muscular cover.

189 Passive, so-called 'forced' rehabilitation by mechanotherapy is indisputably aggressive, so also is massage.

190 Various theories have been formulated: neurogenic, vascular, neurovascular, hormonal and neurovascular, inflammatory, biochemical, etc. with no consensus except that it is triggered by an 'aggressor' in the form of an abnormal autonomic nervous response, the reality of which seems to be confirmed by the influence of treatment orientated towards the sympathetic system.

191 The quote 'you have to want algonemodystrophy to get it' has led it to be called the 'organic neurosis of the locomotor system'.

The bone lesion is diffuse, at both macroscopic and microscopic levels resembling common osteoporosis, characterized by a decrease in the number and thickness of bone trabeculae as well as other features.

Clinical examination

The interview establishes the connection between trauma and the painful incapacity. At the onset the trauma is not always significant; and, since violent trauma itself produces a painful incapacity, it can hide the disease for weeks or months.

The superficial signs trauma rapidly resolve, but the painful incapacity persists or increases, making it possible to detect the disease in the days that follow.

The characteristics of this painful incapacity are: diffuse, lancinating pain radiating upward and downward, acute and sometimes excruciating, continuous at certain periods, paradoxically exacerbated by immobilization and to an even greater extent by a cast. The incapacity may be severe with limping and require crutches.

The examination findings are a knee which is deformed in painless flexion, decreased in volume by muscle wasting[192], hot and red[193], essentially painful and sometimes with acute pain arising from simple touch or the least movement.

Radiological examination

There may be several weeks' lag before radiological symptoms appear[194]. Osteoporosis is characterized by bone rarefaction that is both isolated and spotty. Isolated rarefaction is shown by the lack of involvement of bone contours and joint interlines. Spotty rarefaction produces clear, rounded and well delineated zones that are initially punctiform, but that extend and converge so that all three stages may be juxtaposed on the same x-ray:

(1) The initial or geodic stage has a spotty appearance.

(2) The second or lacunar stage has a flaky, mottled or stippled appearance.

(3) The third or transparent stage occurs more often in the 'glass bone' form than the 'combed' form[195].

Course

The course is extended and can be counted in months or years, but with the certainty of a cure and, as a rule, with no sequelae in the knee[196].

Capsular Retraction

The peripheral, capsular and ligamentous tissue can be shortened by retraction, leading to insufficient stiffness. Only posterolateral retraction will be considered here, because of the major loss of extension that it causes[197].

Pathogenesis

The topography is limited to the middle and particularly the posterior thirds of the lateral (p. 18) and medial (p. 20) peripheral apparatus.

Polymicrotrauma (p. 89) is probably responsible for overexertion of the synovium, resulting in synovitis; the cause is commonly iatrogenic, particularly following surgery for meniscal, capsular and ligamentous surgery and nearly always after unsuitable rehabilitation[198]. 'Synovitis' is a retractile sclerosis[199]: the capsule loses its flexibility and shrinks.

The loss of the resting position (p. 51 and Note 68) is eminently restrictive for the patellofemoral joint[200].

---

192 The contrast is emphasized by the possible appearance of diffuse non pitting oedema in the foot and leg.

193 The hot, red knee can sometimes become cyanotic and cold, thereby reflecting the two phases of a vasomotor reaction that has exceeded its objective.

194 The pitfall of x-ray lag may be compensated by scintigraphy (p. 86): the hyperactive zone is significant because it is both diffuse and uniform, occasionally exceeding the limits of the knee and spreading to the diaphyses and involving the vascular component of the soft tissue.

195 The bone matrix may, in the final stage of diffuse rarefaction, either become indistinct with 'glass bone' appearance or become partially transparent with a coarse 'combed' or fibrillar appearance.

196 The disease does not normally recur.

197 As a rule, anterolateral capsular retraction is not detected from a loss of the last degrees of flexion: in fact, this is a sector of mobility rarely used except by athletes and exceptional acrobatic movements requiring complete flexion.

198 Rehabilitation can be considered irrational if it does not respect the major principles, which are painlessness, basic recovery of passive extension (p. 33 and 34) and subsequently of muscular strength through isometric exercise (p. 53 and Note 72), the recovery of tendon, capsule and ligament vigilance (p. 69 and Note 97), etc.; in fact all 'forced' rehabilitation causing the reappearance of pain or effusion, or proceeding initially with for example, passive flexion exercises will terminate in a reactional 'synovitis', which will cause capsular retraction.

199 The fibroblastic reaction spreading from the synovium toward the capsule invades the space separating the two membranes, constituting retractile capsulitis.

200 The active knee in flexion (p. 56) can recover a precarious equilibrium, but only by paying with an excessive increase in patellar compression of the femur: in fact, the stabilizing muscular force permanently applied by the quadriceps avoids the knee bending under weight-bearing when the line of gravity falls behind the extension-flexion centre.

Clinical examination
The clinical examination is dominated by locking in extension (p. 66).

Opaque arthrography
Opaque arthrography may be significant (p. 81), with resistance to injection and the decrease of the area injected. The resistance is manifested with the last ml of the normal volume of injection, by liquid squirting back when the syringe is removed from the needle. The decrease in the surface area injected appears on the lateral views, in extension and even more in flexion, by the disappearance of the posterior bursae.

Spontaneous course
As a rule, the condition persists[201] if untreated, but resolves with treatment and does not normally recur.

Tendon-muscle lesions

Stress-induced lesions of the extensor apparatus

Pathogenesis reveals two major causes, one common and the other specific.

The common cause for tendon-muscle disease is fatigue and its many aggravating factors, which are particularly insidious in high level athletes[202]. 'General' fatigue is signalled by immediate cramp and contracture the following day, reflecting insufficient metabolic recovery caused by too much competition or inadequate training. Local fatigue reflects periarticular stiffness by reducing tendon-muscle elasticity, a consequence of sports polymicrotraumata (p. 89).

A number of aggravating factors that are usually unapparent or negligible in the non-athlete may sooner or later cause the 'precision mechanism of a champion' to 'freeze up', particularly: disalignment of the tibiofemoral axis and patellar disequilibrium disrupting the lines of force and favouring an unadapted sports discipline; tendon-muscle 'fragility' incurred by adolescents participating in an unbalanced sports activity[203].

Tendon degeneration[204] is a precocious finding in adults who practice sports intensively[205]. Active/passive destabilization in the knee is caused by inadequate surgical repair, rehabilitation in physical therapy, readaptation in training, preparation for competition, recovery in sports effort, the shock wave coming from sudden impact on hard soil, error in a technical manoeuvre, etc.

The specific cause of disease of the extensor apparatus is both anatomical and physiological.

The anterior location of the extensor apparatus predisposes it to contusions. Its function leaves it vulnerable by subjecting it to rotary constraints when the femur and tibia move in opposite directions; the quadriceps tendon depends exclusively on the femur in attaching itself to the patella, which is a 'prisoner' of the trochlea, and the patellar tendon depends essentially on the tibia because it is attached to the anterior tibial tuberosity and cannot be extended.

The extensor apparatus is subject to serious as well as benign tendinomuscular lesions. Rupture of the quadriceps tendon or patellar ligament has to be diagnosed as serious (p. 63 and Note 4) for orthopaedic or surgical treatment to be indicated.

Rupture of the quadriceps tendon QT (p. 24)

This is a partial rupture[206].

Pathogenesis
The pathogenesis is characterized by a disinsertion of the lower rectus femoris RF (p. 23) when

---

201 Persistence beyond the sixth month would particularly arouse fears in arthrosis (p. 84): reactional 'synovitis' will be predisposed by wearing out of the synovium, particularly on the lowest parts, which fill with cartilaginous debris from articular deterioration.

202 The high level athlete is dedicated to high performance and must therefore constantly operate at close to the upper limit of resistance, but at a risk of exceeding his limits and 'breaking down'.

203 Excessive muscle-building, training that neglects endurance essential for recovery and stressing strength that is dominant in the game leads to emphasis on muscular body development with increased power but at the cost of a double handicap, sometimes definitive at maturity: decreased possibility of recovery and wound healing because of vascular insufficiency; establishing a weak point at the tendon-muscle junction because of the disproportion between the enlarging muscle body and the tendon, whose cross-sectional area remains practically unchanged.

204 Tendon degeneration is a histological entity which goes through a series of four types of lesion during its cyclic development: alteration of the fundamental substance; fibrinoid, mucoid or hyalin degeneration; initiation of tendon rupture; inconstant appearance of scar nodules.

205 Intensive sports, professional or semi-professional, cause 'physiological aging' to arrive earlier (p. 114 Note 87) so that tendon degeneration suffers the same fate as cartilage involution in the context of accelerated 'wear'. As a result x-ray findings of arthrosis which are frequent in professional soccer players from age 25 on, can give the impression that the knee has run up a lifetime's 'mileage' during ten or fifteen years of a sports career.

206 The total rupture that strikes elderly subjects is excluded by definition (p. 89).

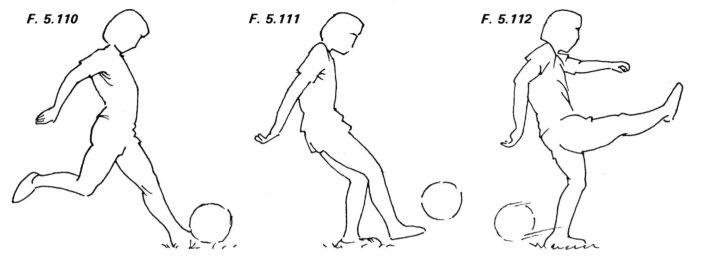

F. 5.110 F. 5.111 F. 5.112

excessive demands are made on the quadriceps[207] (Figures 5.110–5.112).

Clinical examination
The seriousness of the injury can be assessed by asking about the three signs of alarm occurring at the time of the initial accident: 'syncopal' pain, snapping, and total and immediate incapacity (p. 66).

The examination identifies the rupture by morphological and functional signs that are capable of eventually being modified: filling of the transverse groove by the haematoma; the retraction and balling up of the proximal end, which is evident in contraction against resistance; ecchymosis that is often delayed and lopsided (p. 66); reproduction of pain and evaluation of the deficiency by using the muscle evaluation (p. 69).

Special examinations
The condition of the lesion can be precisely indicated by using the combined thermography-ultrasound test (p. 88). Thermography will detect an abnormally cold area; ultrasound sometimes locates an area that is not very dense to ultrasound.

Course
The handicap will be evident during sports activity, and in everyday existence by difficulty in descending stairs. The condition will become inexorably chronic, depending on how long it takes for several factors to occur. These are: the appearance of a fibrous scar causing shortening (p. 70 and Note 41); and the transformation of pooled blood into an 'active' cyst[208], or 'passive' ossification[209].

Rupture of the patellar ligament PL (p. 24)

This may be partial or complete.

Pathogenesis
The condition is caused by straining the patellar ligament[210] through excessive demand on the whole quadriceps[211].

Clinical examination
As a rule, it is easy to differentiate between partial and complete rupture. Complete rupture (p. 63) because of its seriousness, will usually be obvious from the history, but this is not the case with partial rupture.

Examination of the partial rupture will reveal a painful hardening located in the middle of the tendon, close to its patellar insertion. A complete rupture is obvious, with a transverse furrow of the rupture appearing above the high, retracted patella, which is still solidly connected to the quadriceps and with the impossibility of active extension.

---

207 The excessive demand to which the RF is predisposed (p. 57, Notes 84 and 86) is illustrated by the soccer player during the series of three movements involved in making a shot. The first movement involves complete extension of the hip while the RF is stretched at the point of departure by a broad pendular movement that should terminate in flexing the hip (Figure 5.111). The second movement is at the approach to extension of the knee while the RF may be called upon to provide nearly all of the effort (Figure 5.112). The third movement is complete extension of the knee while the RF participates in contraction against resistance in recovering a ball 'on the fly', or an opposing pass or shot (Figure 5.112).

208 The cyst, by playing the role of an artificial bursa in sliding, can work against muscular movement like a 'useless pulley', justifying excision in the athlete.

209 Once the ossification is 'mature', it can be forgotten to the point of no longer handicapping the athlete.

210 The strength of the patellar ligament is related to its inability to stretch (p. 36 and Note 23).

211 Excessive demand on the quadriceps is illustrated by the example of the bicyclist going uphill in a standing position (Figure 5.113): the power of the mobilizing force that increases with extension (p. 57) is abruptly transmitted to each pedal by the patellar ligament, but with the risk of a rupture and occasionally avulsion of point of the patella.

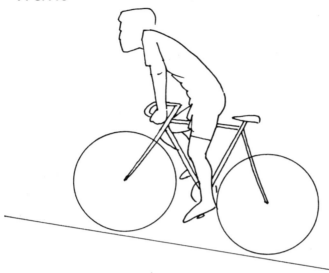

Radiological examination
The lateral views (p. 77 and 80), confirm the complete rupture with an image of high, retracted patella, and occasionally avulsion of the extra-articular point of the patella (p. 11).

Special examinations
Ultrasonic tomography (p. 84) identifies the partial rupture in the form of an empty, fluid image showing a clearly defined fragment[212].

Course
Complete rupture leads to a chronic condition which makes active extension impossible[213], while partial rupture handicaps only athletes.

Benign lesion caused by patellar tendonitis

When a diagnosis of serious conditions is eliminated and before undertaking medical or physical treatment, patellar tendonitis should be considered the cause of the patient's problem.

Pathogenesis
Tendonitis of the insertion implies localization in one or the other of the tendons. The condition has various names such as enthesitis, athlopathy, technopathy, etc, which demonstrate the determining role of sports polymicrotraumata, particularly cycling.

---

212 The transsonic image that is obtained is indirect proof of rupture on the basis of a deep, encysted haematoma.

213 The loss of the compensators is the cause: in fact, complete rupture of the patellar tendon spreads to the tendon-aponeurotic expansions (p. 26) and associates with tears of the patellar retinacula (p. 20 and 22).

Clinical examination
The interview establishes the relationship between an intermittent pain (p. 63) and a specific movement or position in athletes.

The examination reveals pain precisely located by palpation (p. 66) that reproduces isometric contraction and maximum stretching of the extensor apparatus (p. 70).

Radiological examination
X-rays can show tenoperiostitis in the late stage: chronic irritation of the periosteum near the tendon insertion produces a blurred image bristling with osteophytes or microossifications.

Special examinations
They are reassuring in cases of radiating pain where there is no discontinuity in the tendon: thermography and ultrasonic tomography are normal while zero radiography (p. 86) may detect the initial stage of tendonitis.

Course
Sooner or later healing occurs, but the subject must give up sports until this occurs.

Other conditions of tendons

Isolated rupture of a tendon

Apart from a dominant meniscal, capsular and ligamentous lesion, isolated rupture of a tendon is unusual; occurring in the popliteal tendon in posterolateral laxity (p. 99 and 103), the popliteal and biceps tendons in anteroposterolateral laxity (p. 104), and the semimembranous insertion complex in anteroposteromedial laxity (p. 104).

Pure tendonitis

Pure tendonitis is as exceptional except in pes anserinus (p. 28) where tenobursitis is identical to cellulalgia of the medial face of the knee, a condition predominantly occurring in women.

Traumatic liporarthritis (Hoffa's disease)

The cause of this disorder is not clear, but it easily slips into surgeons' operative reports.

Pathogenesis is an inflammation of the fat pad (p. 20), and is of traumatic origin, leading to localized or diffuse hyperplasia.

Clinical examination reveals a painful and bilobate swelling occurring in any part of the patellar ligament.

Radiological examination is normal.

Special examinations give negative results with the exception of xeroradiography (p. 86), which may show the fat pad in a triangular, hypertrophied image, with scattered microcalcifications.

The course is undetermined.

Post-traumatic periarthritis (Pellegrini-Steida syndrome)

This is an ossifying disorder, often related to a neglected sprain.

Pathogenesis
The topographical distribution is usually limited to the medial face of the knee; elective localization is para or supracondylar.

The condition is triggered by direct contact and, in principle, is a sprain resulting from direct violence with medial impact: posterolateral laxity version 2 (p. 103 and Note 59) and anteroposterolateral laxity (p. 104 and Note 66) are therefore also involved.

The typical lesion is independent: the 'kneeing' or kick causes a haematoma to form at the point of medial impact[214]. This forms a new and separate formation that becomes fibrous, cartilaginous and then ossifies.

Clinical and radiological examination
When examining for laxity, there is a risk of limiting oneself to the 'epicondylitis' that monopolizes the clinician's attention in two respects. The initial appearance is pseudo-inflammatory, with swelling, redness, heat and pain, with painless flexion or a painful range of movement. The later appearance is more definitive with the appearance of a true osteoma of the femur, hard and painless, limiting

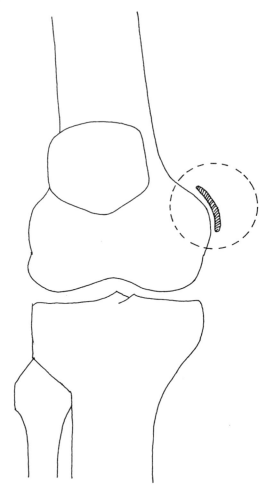

F. 5.114

flexion by interfering with sliding, and showing a suggestive crescent-shaped opacity[215] (Figure 5.114).

Course
There are two possible courses, both of which can be detected radiographically.

(1) Non-stabilized, heterogeneous opacity, with a blurred contour, increasing in volume until it encounters the bone. This cannot be treated surgically.

(2) Stabilized, uniform opacity, with sharp contours, and maintaining the same volume. This is a possible candidate for ablation.

---

214 The lateral impact is more often accompanied by a diffusion of the haematoma which the less 'hermetic' lateral structures favour (p. 18, 27 and 30).

215 The osteoma becomes visible as soon as it is ossified, several weeks or months after the trauma.

Chapter 6

DIAGNOSTIC NOTES

(1) Painful knee (gonalgia) may indicate pain at some distance above or below the knee. This condition requires a complete systematic examination, with particular attention focused on the hip and lumbar spine; in fact, any gonalgia that cannot definitively be attributed to the knee normally indicates pain projected from disorders of the hip and femur or of the L2-L3 or L3-L4 vertebral joints.

(2) Pain in posterolateral laxity (pp. 99, 103) may be insufficiently or inaccurately interpreted. An isolated lesion of the lateral meniscus (p. 89) or tendonitis of the popliteal tendon (p. 141) may monopolize attention and it is possible to be deceived by the 'locking' of the proximal tibiofibular joint (p. 132) or by 'fabellitis' (p. 134).

(3) Pseudo-genu varum may appear to be true genu varum (p. 118), if it has not been verified by correction under two sets of circumstances: pseudo-genu varum of osseous origin occurs in lateral tibial hypertorsion through medial rotation of bone elements (p. 121 and Note 120); pseudo-genu varum of articular origin occurs in genu recurvatum through medial rotation of the tibia under the femur (p. 122 and Note 129).

(4) Pseudo-locking (p. 64 and Note 14) is of reflex origin, which is mostly caused by patellar disequilibrium (pp.119-121 and Note 110; pp. 126 and 127).

(5) 'True' locking (p. 64 and Note 14) is of mechanical origin and is not primarily caused by a meniscal or osteocartilaginous obstacle. Elastic locking in extension is found particularly in the isolated lesion of the medial meniscus, but in an unapparent or unpredictable form that makes it an inconstant sign (p. 87). It can be caused by posterolateral capsular retraction (p. 137) following an inadequately treated or untreated sprain, and can be simulated by the cellular, tendon and muscle pain syndrome of a valgus of spinal origin confirmed by the instantaneous and astonishing result of lumbar massage focused on L3-L4.

(6) A history of a 'swollen knee' in the findings of a haemarthrosis can mean three different things within the limited context of joint pathology: the isolated lesion of the anterior cruciate ligament (pp. 95 and 101), lateral luxation of the patella (p. 128) and post-traumatic osteochondral lesions (p. 128).

(7) Ecchymosis, if it has not been proved abarticular and caused by 'kneeing', a kick or the 'snapping' of a tendinomuscular structure, can be considered equivalent to a haemarthrosis (p. 66) but can be missed in the absence of knee swelling.

(8) Anterior drawer sign—rotation O may be imitated by a spontaneous posterior drawer sign maintained by leg weight (pp. 68, 71).

(9) Anterior and posterior drawer sign—rotation O, occurring in the presence of anteroposterolateral laxity (p. 104) or anteroposteromedial laxity (p. 106), including a lesion of both the ACL and the PCL, are not precise because it is impossible to determine the neutral position. The radiodynamic drawer sign is more determinant, with the advantage of having comparative x-rays to confirm them (p. 76).

(10) Pivot shift test is pathognomonic of a lesion of the anterior cruciate ligament (p. 95) but with two reservations related to the isolated lesion (p. 101, 102): the test may be negative in any partial lesion of the ACL, delayed degeneration and precocious disinsertion or tearing; it may be positive in the absence of any sensation of instability, with the risk of subsequent decompensation of a united and inseparable functional unit.

(11) Patella bipartita, the most frequent patellar dysplasia, may become painful through a chance trauma directed toward the superior lateral corner of the patella. The clinical picture is of superior lateral separation, usually bilateral, rounded, uniform, with a clear and regular contour confirming its constitutional origin in relation to osteonecrosis (p. 129), a foreign body, avulsion, or ossification of the ligament.

(12) Fracture of the patella may occur as an alternative to total rupture of the patellar tendon, acompanied by avulsion of the extra-articular point of the patella (p. 139).

(13) Radiological findings in lateral luxation of the patella followed by reduction may be normal; 'true' luxation of a patella that is normally balanced and accompanied at least by a pure condylar fracture may remain undetected (p. 118).

(14) Fracture of the head of the fibula is possible if direct violence occurs with a point of impact on the

posterolateral facet of the flexed knee (p. 98 and Note 38), possibly hiding a serious sprain that results in anteromedial laxity.

(15) Post-traumatic periarthritis with stabilized ossification (p. 141) can be confused with the pseudo-arthrosis of ligamentous and periosteal avulsion of the tibial collateral ligament.

(16) Partial degeneration of the ACL clinging to and being nourished by another structure (p. 95) may be consolidated through a hypertrophic scar formation process with suspended ossification appearing in the intercondylar notch, to the point of imposing osteochondromatosis (p. 114 et seq).

(17) Opacification of the popliteal tendon in arthrography (p. 81) may be confused with the normally distinct images of a vertical tear of the posterior horn of the lateral meniscus (p. 89).

(18) Isolated meniscal lesions do exist (p. 87 et seq), but rarely: in fact the meniscal lesion is most often 'third member of the party' in a meniscal, capsular and ligamentous lesion (p. 93 et seq).

(19) Osteochondral lesions of frontal patellar disequilibrium (p. 118 et seq) or sagittal disequilibrium (p. 126 et seq), post-traumatic chondromalacia of the patella (p. 128), etc. may occur as an alternative to partial rupture of the patellar ligament (p. 139); the patellar ligament, in its turn, may manifest patellar tendonitis (p. 140) or traumatic lipoarthritis (p. 141).

(20) A hyperactive site of circumscribed osteonecrosis in the adolescent (p. 130 and Note 160) may be missed, and can be overlaid by normal hyperfixation at the age of cartilage conjugation: in this type of case, comparative studies should demonstrate asymmetry in tracer fixation.

(21) Deep bursitis and popliteal cysts (p. 133) should be differentiated from rampant and expanding aneurisms, the painful and hardened cord of deep venous thrombosis, muscular hypertrophy, etc.

(22) Post-traumatic algoneurodystrophy (p. 136) in its initial infraradiological phase, may suggest rheumatoid or microbial monoarthritis.

(23) Traumatic lipoarthritis (p 141) is meaningful only in terms of an iatrogenic origin: introduction of a corticoid in suspension by anterior route using too short a needle, may trigger an inflammatory reaction in the fat pad.

Abbreviations

Abd Abduction
ACL Anterior cruciate ligament
AD Anterior drawer
Add Adduction
ADMR Anterior drawer—medial rotation
ADLR Anterior drawer—lateral rotation
ADRO Anterior drawer—RO
AHLM Anterior horn of the lateral meniscus
AHMM Anterior horn of the medial meniscus
ALL Anterolateral laxity
AM Active mobility
AM Adductor magnus
AML Anteromedial laxity
AP Anteposition
APL Arcuate popliteal ligament
APLL Anteroposterolateral laxity
APML Anteroposteromedial laxity
AS Active stability
ASIT Anterior superior iliac tubercule
ASL Anterior subluxation
ATF Anterior thrust of the femur
ATFg Anterior thrust of the femur—gravity component

ATFm Anterior thrust of the femur—muscular component
ATrT Force of anterior traction of the tibia
ATT Anterior tibial tuberosity

B Biceps muscle
BI Bone interline
BT Big Toe test
BTd Biceps tendon

c Functional centre of the patella
Cap Capsule
CAT Computerised axial tomography
CGL Crossed global laxity
CI Cartilage interline
COM Angle of lateral tibial torsion
COT Angle of tibiofemoral divergence
CPN Common peroneal nerve

d Distance
DE Drawer-extension

F Anatomical axis of the femur
Fa Fabella
FCL-L Fibular collateral ligament (long)

FCL-S Fibular collateral ligament (short)
FL Fascia lata
Fo Forward
FOT Angle of alignment or disalignment of the anatomical axes
FP Fat pad
F3P 3rd facet of the patella

G Gastrocnemius
GAL Global anterior laxity
GCL Global crossed laxity
GFx Genu flexum
GLL Global lateral laxity
GlM Gluteus muscles
Gr Gravity or weight-bearing
GrM Gracilis muscle
GRv Genu recurvatum
GSB Gastrocnemio-semimembranous bursa
GVl Genu valgum
GVr Genu varum

H Horizontal
HE Hyperextension
HM Hamstring muscles

ICN Intercondylar notch
IE Intercondylar eminence
IF Infrapatellar fold
IL ACL Isolated lesion of the anterior cruciate ligament
IL PCL Isolated lesion of the posterior cruciate ligament
IO Interline opening
ITA Iliotibial aponeurosis
ITB Iliotibial band

L Lateral
LB Long head of the biceps
LBC Lateral back corner
LC Lateral constraints
LDM Lateral dynamic mooring
LEF Lateral epicondyle of the femur
LFc Lateral front corner
LFC Lateral femoral condyle
LFL Lateral femoropatellar ligament
LFT Lateral facet of the trochlea
LFP Lateral facet of the patella
LG Lateral gastrocnemius
LHR Lateral hyper-rotation
LI Lateral interline
LIMS Lateral intermuscular septum
LM Lateral meniscus
LMPL Lateral meniscopatellar ligament
LO Lateral opening
LPC Lateral posterior capsule
LPR Lateral patellar retinaculum
LR Lateral rotation
LRF Force of lateral rotation of the femur
LRT Lateral rotation of the tibia under the femur
LSL Lateral subluxation
LTC Lateral tibial condyle
LTP Force of lateral translation of the patella
LTT Lateral tibial tuberosity

M Bimalleolar axis
M Medial
MA Mechanical axis of the tibiofemoral
MBC Medial back corner
MDM Medial dynamic mooring
ME Medial epicondyle of the femur
MF Meniscofemoral bundle
MFC Medial femoral condyle
MFL Medial femoropatellar ligament
MFP Medial facet of the patella
MFT Medial facet of the trochlea
MG Medial gastrocnemius
MGB Medial gastrocnemius bursa
MHR Medial hyper-rotation
MI Medial interline
MIMS Medial intermuscular septum
MM Medial meniscus
MMPL Medial meniscopatellar ligament
MO Medial opening
MOC Angle of talus-calcaneus divergence

MPC Medial posterior capsule
MPR Medial patellar retinaculum
MR Medial rotation
MRT Force of medial rotation of the tibia
MSLM Middle segment of the lateral meniscus
MSMM Middle segment of the medial meniscus
MTB Meniscotibial bundle
MTC Medial tibial condyle
MTT Medial tibial tubercle
MTTy Medial tibial tuberosity
MW Meniscal wall

N Normal
NLR Necessary lateral rotation
NMR Necessary medial rotation

O Axis of extension–flexion
O Axis of rotation
OPL Oblique popliteal ligament

P Popliteal muscle
P Angle of opening of the patella
PA Pes anserinus
PC Posterior constraints
PCF Patellar compression of femur
PCL Posterior cruciate ligament
PC-PCL Torque posterior constraints—posterior cruciate ligament
PD Posterior drawer
PDLR Posterior drawer—lateral rotation
PDMR Posterior drawer—medial rotation
PDRO Posterior drawer—rotation O
PH Popliteal hiatus
PHLM Posterior horn of the lateral meniscus
PHMM Posterior horn of the medial meniscus
PL Posterior laxity
PLg Patellar ligament
PLL Posterolateral laxity
PMFL Posterior meniscofemoral ligament
PML Posteromedial laxity
PMT Posterior border of the medial tibial condyle
POC Angle of anteversion of the neck of the femur
POL Posterior oblique ligament
POM Angle of torsion of the lower limb
PPB Prepatellar bursa
Pr Retroposition
PS Pivot shift
PSL
PT Popliteal tendon
PTB Pretibial bursa
PTrT Force of posterior traction of the tibia

Pv Pelvis

Q Quadriceps muscle
Q-ACL Torque quadriceps—anterior cruciate ligament
QCR Angle of alignment or disalignment of the extensor apparatus
QT Quadriceps tendon

R Rear
RO Rotation zero
RcT Recurrent tendon
RF Rectus femoris
RfT Reflected tendon
Rl Rolling
RP Retroposition
RPF Retropatellar fold
RPS Reverse pivot shift
RxD Radiodynamic drawer
RxO Radiodynamic opening

Sar Sartorius muscle
SB Short head of the biceps
Sl Sliding
SM Semimembranous muscle
SPF Suprapatellar fold
SQSB Subquadricipital serous bursa
ST Semitendinous muscle
StT Straight tendon
Syn Synovium

T Anatomical axis of the tibia
T̂ Angle of opening of the trochlea
TA
TCL Tibial collateral ligament
TICS Tibial intercondylar space
TL Transverse ligament of the knee
TLTC Top of the lateral tibial condyle
TOM Angle of lateral tibial torsion
TT Trochlear throat

V Vertical
VAD Voluntary anterior drawer sign
VI Vastus intermedius
VL Vastus lateralis muscle
Vl Valgus
VlE Valgus—extension
VlLR Valgus—lateral rotation
VlMR Valgus—medial rotation
VM Vastus medialis muscle
VML Vastus medialis muscle (longitudinal)
VMO Vastus medialis muscle (oblique)
VPD Voluntary posterior drawer sign
Vr Varus
VrE Varus—extension
VrLR Varus—lateral rotation
VrMR Varus—medial rotation